CBD

for Your
Health, Mind
& Spirit

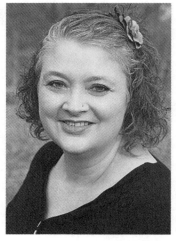

About the Author

Kerri Connor has been practicing her craft for over thirty-five years and has run an eclectic Pagan family group, The Gathering Grove, since 2003.

She is a frequent contributor to Llewellyn annuals and is the author of *Wake, Bake & Meditate: Take Your Spiritual Practice to a Higher Level with Cannabis* and *420 Meditations*. Kerri runs The Spiral Labyrinth, a mini spiritual retreat, at her home in Ringwood, IL.

ADVICE, RECIPES, AND MEDITATIONS
to Alleviate Ailments
& Connect *to* Spirit

CBD

for Your
Health, Mind
& Spirit

KERRI CONNOR
With Cheryl Cryer

Llewellyn Publications
Woodbury, Minnesota

FIRST EDITION
First Printing, 2022

Book design by Christine Ha
Cover design by Shira Atakpu

Llewellyn Publications is a registered trademark of Llewellyn Worldwide Ltd.

Library of Congress Cataloging-in-Publication Data
Names: Connor, Kerri, author.
Title: CBD for your health, mind & spirit : advice, recipes, and
 meditations to alleviate ailments & connect to spirit / Kerri Connor.
Other titles: CBD for your health, mind and spirit
Description: First edition. | Woodbury, Minnesota : Llewellyn Worldwide,
 Ltd, [2022] | Includes bibliographical references. | Summary: "CBD is
 one of the most versatile and healing plant compounds in existence, and
 Kerri Connor explains what CBD can do, where to buy it, and how to use
 it. This book includes tips for working with CBD for healing and
 wellness of humans and pets and integrating CBD into spiritual
 practice"—Provided by publisher.
Identifiers: LCCN 2021060786 (print) | LCCN 2021060787 (ebook) | ISBN
 9780738767659 (paperback) | ISBN 9780738767758 (ebook)
Subjects: LCSH: Cannabis—Therapeutic use. | Cannabinoids—Therapeutic use.
Classification: LCC RM666.C266 C658 2022 (print) | LCC RM666.C266 (ebook)
 | DDC 615.7/827—dc23/eng/20211220
LC record available at https://lccn.loc.gov/2021060786
LC ebook record available at https://lccn.loc.gov/2021060787

Llewellyn Worldwide Ltd. does not participate in, endorse, or have any authority or responsibility concerning private business transactions between our authors and the public.

All mail addressed to the author is forwarded but the publisher cannot, unless specifically instructed by the author, give out an address or phone number.

Any internet references contained in this work are current at publication time, but the publisher cannot guarantee that a specific location will continue to be maintained. Please refer to the publisher's website for links to authors' websites and other sources.

Llewellyn Publications
A Division of Llewellyn Worldwide Ltd.
2143 Wooddale Drive
Woodbury, MN 55125-2989
www.llewellyn.com

Printed in the United States of America

For Fat Sam and Xena

Disclaimer

Using, distributing, or selling cannabis is a federal crime and may be illegal in your state or local vicinity. It is your responsibility to understand all laws pertaining to the possession or use of cannabis. Neither the author nor the publishers are accountable for consequences derived from the possession or use thereof. Always seek the advice of a qualified health provider regarding medical questions. This book is not a substitute for medical advice. CBD may counteract certain medications, including those used to treat blood pressure, blood clots, and thyroid, liver, and heart issues. In some medications such as antidepressants, it may increase the effects. Consult with your doctor before using CBD to ensure it is safe for you.

Contents

Chapter 6

The Mind   113

Chapter 7

The Spirit   137

Introduction

You are curious about CBD. You've heard about it, you've seen it in stores and on signs, and you know people who rave about it. But you aren't sure what it can do for you, where to buy it, or how to use it. You may have friends swear by it to help their ailments, but since you don't have the same condition, you don't know how it could help you or even if it could help you. Maybe you have even tried a CBD oil once and were put off by the taste, or the dosage you tried didn't have any effect. You have heard so much good about it; you want to give it a serious try by incorporating it into your life and diet. You want to learn how it can help you and maybe even someday replace your prescribed pharmaceuticals (under a doctor's care, of course). This book is here to help answer all your questions and get you started on the right path to a relationship with one of the most versatile and healing plants in existence: cannabis (also known as hemp). CBD stands for *cannabidiol*, one of hundreds of cannabinoids, which come from the cannabis plant. It is a chemical compound different from THC. CBD may be legally sold with up to 0.3 percent THC in it, which allows relief for those who live in areas where medicinal cannabis is illegal or those who want help but not the side effects of THC. It is important to point out, this amount of THC is untraceable in the body and therefore will not have any real effects on the body or mind. My friend Cheryl Cryer, who owns and operates CryBaby CBD, and I collaborated on this book to inform you what CBD is, what it does, how it helps, and how to use it.

In the beginning of this book, we will take a journey to learn some brief history to show us the truth about hemp, including how it came to America. After we learn the history, we will move on to learn about the science, including the endocannabinoid system and how CBD and other cannabinoids are designed to work with your body.

Of course, we will learn about dosing—how to do it and where to start. Microdosing is all the rage and allows the body to keep CBD levels elevated continuously, which means the effects won't wear off. Constantly replenishing the CBD in your system with microdosing keeps you in a stable state of healing.

Not only does the science teach how CBD works, but it also verifies what is a safe product and what is not. The science chapter will also introduce you to terpenes and explain how terpenes can work with CBD (or THC) to produce more intense, stronger effects.

Once we know the history and science, we can start exploring all the many options available to you in how you can use CBD. It comes in many different forms—flower, concentrates, powders, oil—and this can be quite confusing to people who are new to it. Big tip: other than companies wanting to make money, one reason there are so many of them is to make it easier to find what works best for you. Using CBD is trial and error. There is no real other way to do it. Knowing what you are working with is paramount to your success. Educating yourself on what you are using is critical. You have already started by reading this book, but there is more research and trial and error to be done.

In "The Body" chapter, we will share recipes for different ways of using CBD both topically and internally to help heal your physical body. We can use CBD for many reasons because there is a broad category of ailments it helps. The most common issues for using CBD are to fight pain and anxiety. Inflammation, digestive issues, seizures, and even acne can all be treated with CBD. Teas and oils are some of my favorite ways to administer CBD. They are easy to make at home and are designed to work with the terpenes of the other ingredients. You can always take a dropper full of CBD or pop a capsule in your mouth, but there are ways to build a real relationship with CBD to help you complete the body-mind connection. Using the given recipes will help you build the connection and allow you to turn this practice into a part of your spirituality. When you put more effort into what you do, when you pay more attention to what you do, when you have reverence for what you work with and understand the history and science behind it, you build the body-mind-spirit connection. The CBD you work with almost takes on a persona of its own. You learn to respect the plant and how well it works with your body.

In the chapter "The Mind," we take on matters that can be treated with CBD such as anxiety and insomnia. We will share recipes and tips in this chapter to help relieve some of those issues. They will help put you into a better place mentally and help you relax at the end of the day. A better night of sleep is on the way.

We move on finally to the chapter on "The Spirit," which contains meditations, affirmations, blessings, and all kinds of tips and hints on ways you can turn your CBD use into a daily spiritual experience. By working on being present in your own body, learning to give it the attention it deserves, and how CBD plays a role, you can make the body-mind-spirit connection complete.

Finally, we will finish up with some information on pets, because yes, pets have an endocannabinoid system, which works with CBD too. We now have a way to help our furry, feathered, and other friends deal with pain, anxiety, and other issues in an all-natural way. The things CBD does for humans, it does for other animals. While it does not replace trips to the vet, you may find its use makes those vet appointments far easier for your beloved friend.

Throughout this book, we will sprinkle in firsthand accounts from Cheryl and myself along with several of Cheryl's clients on how CBD has been beneficial for them. More and more, science is showing us what other cultures believed and trusted in for many of thousands of years. With this scientific proof, it is extremely difficult to try to deny how amazing the cannabis/hemp family of plants really is.

Cheryl and I have come to CBD from two different beginnings and from different backgrounds, but we have both benefitted greatly from having CBD in our lives. Cheryl was tired of poor results and awful side effects from pharmaceuticals and began looking for alternatives. She initially found CBD to help with insomnia but continued an all-natural wellness path, immersed herself in learning everything she could on natural healing, and was completely off all prescription medications within two years. She loved the results so much, she wanted to help others. She took her MBA and over twenty years of business experience and opened CryBaby CBD. Cheryl spent over ten years teaching, and this comes through with the way she educates her clients. (Since you may wonder about the name "CryBaby," let me point out, Cheryl is a Roller Derby queen, so don't let the name fool you!)

Her company, CryBaby CBD, is registered with the Illinois Department of Agriculture, and they obtain their high-quality, full-spectrum hemp oil from a US Hemp Authority certified farm and processor. This certification ensures they are getting the best in purity, potency, and transparency. When we talk about the science of CBD in chapter 2, this certification is how you know you are getting what you are paying for and the product is safe. Farms and processors must meet stringent regulations to be certified.

While going through my cancer treatments and a subsequent life-threatening infection, I began using cannabis daily to relieve pain. I had already learned opioids didn't help, and I wasn't about to start taking something again I knew would have no effect on pain but would affect my brain and my liver. I wanted to try cannabis for pain, as I'd had positive results with other natural alternative remedies, which, honestly, surprised me. I had smoked a little as a teenager but hadn't touched cannabis in well over a decade when I decided I needed to at least give it a shot. I had friends with medical cards through our state, and they all recommended I try it. When the pain became unbearable and I could no longer sleep, I finally decided to give it a chance. When it worked immediately, I wished I hadn't waited so long to try it. Since then, I have studied and learned as much as I can about cannabis. With new information constantly available, it can be difficult to keep up with it all. For me, it was a lifesaver.

Now, I use CBD concentrates, gummies, bath salts, balms, massage oils, flower, and more along with my cannabis to help with my autoimmune disorders.

I first began using CBD as a substitute for my regular daily cannabis when I took a trip to New Orleans for Mardi Gras and was unable to legally smoke my medicine there. My first day, I picked up a bottle of 500 mg CBD and was a bit surprised by how well it helped me keep the pain at bay. We did so much walking during the week, there is no way I could have been completely pain free, but I could honestly say the CBD did help. It didn't take away all the pain like pure cannabis did for me, but it did make it far more bearable and put the fires out in my inflamed joints. It was far better at fighting the inflammation than I had expected. It was then I decided to keep some on hand for those days when I am in a flare and need an extra boost.

Eventually, I learned adding in CBD with microdosing combined with my cannabis is usually enough to keep the pain away on a daily basis. Some days are still bad days, though, and an even stronger boost is needed. I used to feel like I lived in a constant flare. Even with all the medications I was on, my autoimmune issues were not under control. I do still have flares, but instead of feeling like I'm in one massive one all the time, it happens for a few days every few months.

Each person will have a different story, but we find many similarities between them. Those turning to CBD have often been disappointed by other medications not working the way they are intended, or they are fed up with the absolutely awful, life-dulling side effects.

The Western world has slowly been learning Eastern medicine does work in many situations, and the use of hemp and cannabis as a medicine is definitely an Eastern tradition. It is a far more natural approach, and you cannot get much more natural than consuming a plant.

It is difficult for me still to this day to fathom how much a plant has changed me. It has changed my physical life, making it possible for me to do things I couldn't do for many years. CBD also gave Cheryl a new life with a new career owning her own CBD company. It's a big change going from a large company working for others to starting your own business and overseeing everything. Cheryl's business is growing and expanding.

I hope CBD can do for you at least a small part of what it has done for Cheryl and me, because if it does, it means it will have changed your life in some positive way. Thirty years ago, I never would have thought I would see myself get all excited over a plant. But what this plant has done for me was not only lifesaving but also life altering. My life is far better off, and I hope yours will be too.

CHAPTER 1

The History of Hemp: Following the Evidence

O ur first lesson begins right now with what exactly hemp is. I will use the words *cannabis* and *hemp* interchangeably because hemp is simply a type of cannabis. Specifically, hemp is *Cannabis sativa* in which the THC level is below 0.3 percent. If the THC level goes above 0.3 percent, it is no longer considered "hemp" and is instead *"Cannabis sativa"* and therefore a federal crime. Yes, seriously. With how the current federal laws read in 2020 while writing this book, this is the difference between legal and illegal. This is the only difference between what we call *hemp* and what we call *cannabis*. Hemp crops coming in with a higher percentage of THC must be destroyed. This legal distinction between hemp and *Cannabis sativa* was established by the United States Agricultural Act of 2014. According to the

United States government, the only thing making it hemp and not cannabis is the THC level.

It is important to point out that hundreds of different strains fall under the *Cannabis sativa* umbrella. Some are bred to be high in THC, some low. Some are bred to be high in CBD, some low. Even though there are differences in strains, the overall plant family they belong to is *Cannabis sativa*, so in this book I will often refer to it simply as cannabis and not just hemp. Cannabis is the scientific name. Hemp is the name we give it when we don't want it to be associated with the cannabis that can make you high. All the same family, all the same plant—just different breeds.

Therefore, if we are going to discuss the history of CBD, we must discuss the history of cannabis since it is where CBD comes from. The history of CBD begins thousands of years before evidence of cannabidiol (CBD) or distinctions based on THC levels ever existed. There are many books available on the market specifically about the history of hemp, so we will only go over a quick breakdown here with the most important events. Be sure to check the bibliography if you are interested in reading more about the history of cannabis and hemp. If we want this plant to help us understand our journey, we must give it the same consideration and work to understand the journey it has taken.

Primal Roots

Ancient peoples throughout the world used cannabis in many ways. It was a food, a fiber, a medicine, and an entheogen. While these people didn't understand cannabinoids, much less specific ones such as CBD or THC, they did know these plants were essential to survival and able to provide relief for a variety of ailments. Mark Ferrara tells us in *Sacred Bliss: A Spiritual History of Cannabis*, "Cannabis use in India precedes the advent of written record keeping."[1] It has been used for thousands and thousands of years.

The cannabis from India and other Asian countries was what we now call *Cannabis indica*. Indica plants are generally a meter shorter than their sativa cousins and have a bushy appearance. Indica strains produce euphoric, happy, restful, peaceful effects from a high. Sativa strains are more energizing, but both types may contain CBD. Combine all these characteristics with other properties of the plant and you get a lean, green, healing machine—which is precisely why ancient civilizations used it for so many purposes.

The Hindu Vedas, written in approximately 1100 BCE, said the god Shiva gave *bhang* (cannabis) to the people for their enjoyment.[2] While they did enjoy smoking cannabis, they also benefitted from eating the seeds. Bhang was used

....

1. Mark S. Ferrara, *Sacred Bliss: A Spiritual History of Cannabis* (Lanham, MD: Rowman & Littlefield, 2018), 13.

2. Martin Booth, *Cannabis: A History* (Transworld Digital, 2011), 24.

as a food source, a medicine, and an entheogen. From India, the use of cannabis travelled to China through trade.

One of the earliest documented uses of cannabis came in the form of pottery decorated with a hemp-made cord. The pottery was found in Yangmingshan in Taiwan and is dated between 10,000 and 3000 BCE.[3] Even if we take the middle ground there and say it's 6000 BCE, this means the people of the time already knew enough about the plant to be able to weave it into rope. This shows us its history goes even further back.

Several Chinese documents, including an agricultural record written in 1600 BCE, identified hemp as a major crop.[4] This shows cannabis was already being cultivated thousands of years ago. Use of the plant growing in the wild and being foraged goes back much further. While the Chinese cultivated cannabis, the people of India and the surrounding mountains were able to walk out into nature and pick it for themselves. They had no need to cultivate it at the time, as they knew where in the wild it grew. When the Chinese began using cannabis in different forms, they quickly moved to cultivating it in order to have a steady supply they did not have to go to others for. Their demand had quickly outpaced the supply.

....

3. Booth, *Cannabis: A History*, 20.

4. Booth, *Cannabis: A History*, 21.

The use of cannabis spread by fishermen, sailors, and other traders from China to other countries. As different areas adopted the use of the plant, different names became prevalent for it. Zoroastrians in the seventh century BCE called it *haoma* or *bhanga*. In India it has been known as bhang or *soma* for centuries.[5] Today, cannabis goes by many names and slang terms, some used more in certain geographical areas than in others.

As religions changed, splintered, and evolved, some aspects dropped off, while others were retained. The consumption of cannabis has been retained through many different religious changes and travels. When the rise of Islam absorbed Zoroastrianism, they took on the use of cannabis, particularly in the Persian Sufi sects.[6]

The Aryan people, who invaded northern India, took the knowledge of cannabis with them and spread it wherever they went. By 1500 BCE, this spread the use of cannabis throughout "Persia, Asia Minor, Greece, the Balkans, Germany and eastern France."[7] Later, around 800 BCE, a second group of Aryans, known as Scythians—another conquering group—brought cannabis into Israel, Jordan, and Syria.

....

5. Chris Bennett, "Venerable Traditions: A Brief History of the Ritual and Religious Use of Cannabis," in *Cannabis and Spirituality: An Explorer's Guide to an Ancient Plant Spirit Ally*, ed. by Stephen Gray (Rochester, VT: Park Street Press, 2016), 43.

6. Ferrara, *Sacred Bliss*, 37.

7. Booth, *Cannabis: A History*, 27.

The Scythians were documented as using cannabis by the fifth century BCE Greek historian Herodotus of Halicarnassus. He documented the Scythians using cannabis in a sauna-like setting, throwing flower buds onto hot stones while sitting in covered pits. Russian archaeological excavations in 1929 and 1993 uncovered different Scythian artifacts including smoking pipes, stored cannabis seeds, hemp clothing, and even a container of cannabis. What had once been used by one group of people in one geographic area had already travelled thousands of miles and passed through the hands of many different cultures.[8]

According to the website the Ministry of Hemp, hemp paper mills originated in China and the Middle East in the 700s BCE, showing even ancient civilizations were able to see it was beneficial in many ways.[9]

In approximately 70 CE, Greek doctor Pedanius Dioscorides published the book *De Materia Medica* (*On Medical Matters*). This book contained information on *kannabis emeros* and *kannabis agria* (male and female plants), which stated the plant could be used to make rope and to treat earaches. Oddly, nothing was mentioned about it having a psychoactive effect. Later, in 160 CE, another Greek doctor, Claudius Galen, reported hemp cakes could give a person a

....

8. Booth, *Cannabis: A History*, 27–29.

9. "World Timeline of Hemp," Ministry of Hemp, accessed July 9, 2020, https://ministryofhemp.com/hemp/history/.

"feeling of wellbeing but, taken to excess, they led to intoxication, dehydration and impotence."[10]

For hundreds of years, the use of cannabis spread and grew through trade and travels. While some cultures used it to smoke for health or spiritual reasons, other cultures used it for its fibers. Many cultures used it for all its benefits.

Essential Commodity

Over the centuries, hemp, generally in the form of *Cannabis sativa*, became an extremely important crop. The Venetian Republic industrialized hemp, using it to outfit boats with sails and strong ropes and to produce fine linen. The sails they produced allowed for longer, farther trips, increasing their trade and influence from the eleventh through seventeenth centuries.[11]

In 1544, hemp was in such demand, King Henry VIII fined farmers who did not grow it. Hemp crops were essential for ropes, nets, and sails to outfit the British Navy. While the British invented machines to help with the manufacturing process, space for growing hemp was limited, and so King Henry, followed by Queen Elizabeth, fined farmers who did not grow it. The payment for hemp was cheap though, and therefore it wasn't financially beneficial for farmers to be hemp cultivators. After defeating the Spanish Armada, the

....

10. Booth, *Cannabis: A History*, 31.

11. Robert Deitch, *Hemp: American History Revisited: The Plant with a Divided History* (New York: Algora Pub., 2003), 13.

need for hemp was so great in Britain, the Crown turned to Russia to import what was needed.[12] While Britain had the technology, they simply did not have the land to grow as much hemp as was needed. By 1633, 97 percent of Britain's hemp was being imported from Russia. The British knew they needed to find land to grow their own.[13]

Hemp Travels to the Colonies

You may have been taught in school the main reason people came to the colonies was for religious freedom—at least I know back in my day we were. This isn't the whole truth, though. Britain needed land for growing hemp, and they found it. Though the first expedition, known as Roanoke, didn't succeed in surviving, the Jamestown colony did. In 1611, England sent orders to Jamestown to begin growing hemp. In 1619, King James I ordered each colonist who owned property to grow one hundred hemp plants to send back to Britain. As more people immigrated and more colonies appeared, cultivation of hemp moved into the Carolinas and Kentucky areas. Immigrants came from places other than Britain (the Dutch and French), settling in different areas, but they, too, also grew hemp.[14]

As shipbuilding began growing on the northeastern coast, more of the hemp grown in the colonies stayed in the colonies than was being exported back to Britain. By 1630,

....

12. Booth, *Cannabis: A History*, 37.

13. Deitch, *Hemp: American History Revisited*, 13.

14. Deitch, *Hemp: American History Revisited*, 16.

hemp was clothing at least half of the population. In 1637, the General Assembly of Connecticut mandated all families must grow hemp; in 1639, Massachusetts did too.[15]

Virginia enticed hemp dressers from Scandinavia and Poland to come to the colonies by offering them ten guineas. Virginia also made taxes payable with flax, tar, and hemp. According to Booth, "In 1682, Virginia made hemp legal tender in the paying off of up to a quarter of a farmer's debts."[16] I must say, I really wish I could pay off my taxes today by growing hemp or cannabis. I would be more than happy to comply if I had enough for myself too!

By the early 1700s, most colonies had some sort of mandates to encourage the cultivation of hemp. Those that did not mandate it, offered premium prices for crops. One of the problems growing between Britain and the colonies had to do with hemp. While the colonies had to export raw hemp back to Britain, they were also banned from spinning and weaving the hemp themselves, having to buy the final products from Britain too. Basically, they grew hemp, shipped hemp, the millers in Britain would process the hemp, spin the fibers into threads, and weave the threads into materials to be used in other products or sold as material, and then this would be shipped from Britain back to the colonists to purchase. Even with the bans, a spinning

....
15. Booth, *Cannabis: A History*, 40.
16. Booth, *Cannabis: A History*, 40.

industry emerged. (Yes—the colonies revolted against Britain by spinning their own hemp!) When Irish spinners and weavers began immigrating in 1718, the textile industry in the colonies took off. By the time the Revolution came about, the colonies were self-sufficient in hemp and textiles, and exported overages to France.[17]

Sadly, this information is often left out when schools teach the history of America. The importance of hemp in colonizing America was astronomical. In order to eliminate so much reliance on Russia, Britain needed hemp to be grown in the colonies, and it was. Hemp was vital for civilization at the time, as it fulfilled so many needs. It was necessary for ships (strong sails and ropes), which made trade and battles possible—and winnable. It was used for its fibers for clothing (and in the late 1700s—paper). It played a vital role in the expansion of the colonies. The more immigrants came to the colonies, the more hemp was needed. The more it was needed, the less the colonists were willing to work for the benefit of Britain over their own possible benefits, and so the textile industry was born out of rebellion.

In the years leading up to the War of Independence, hemp began being used to make paper. After the American Revolution, hemp became a currency as the different colonies each had their own currencies, which were then left

....
17. Booth, *Cannabis: A History*, 41.

worthless with the introduction of a federal monetary system. Hemp, however, had value throughout the Union.[18]

Cannabis and the Founding Fathers

Before we move on, let's take a quick look at what the founding fathers of the United States thought about cannabis. Not only did they grow and use hemp for fibers, but they also grew and used actual cannabis for medicinal and recreational purposes. The diary of George Washington, the nation's first president, shows he grew his cannabis in a different location than his hemp, and with the cannabis plants, he was focused on the female ones. It is the female plant that contains THC in its buds. It is believed he may have used cannabis to help alleviate tooth pain. Thomas Jefferson, the third president of the United States of America, and one of the authors of the Declaration of Independence, grew cannabis and used it to help treat migraines. All in all, a total of eight United States presidents were known to use cannabis in the early years of our country. The other six were James Madison, James Monroe, Andrew Jackson, Zachary Taylor, Franklin Pierce, and Abraham Lincoln.[19]

Slavery, Eli Whitney, and a Changing Tide

Once slavery came to the colonies, it was used in farming both hemp and cotton. While cotton was an alternative to hemp, the fibers produced were not as strong, and so

....

18. Booth, *Cannabis: A History*, 42.

19. Deitch, *Hemp: American History Revisited*, 25–26.

cotton was not ideal for things like rope and sails, but better for clothing and other material. In 1793, Eli Whitney invented the cotton gin. The cotton "gin" (engine) was able to quickly separate cotton fibers from the seeds, allowing for fast processing. This, combined with slave labor, made cotton cheap.[20] Though slaves did farm hemp, there were not nearly as many working with hemp crops as there were in the cotton fields. By the 1860 census, there were close to four million slaves in the United States, most of them obviously in the South. On April 15, 1861, the Civil War began. Things would never be the same for hemp again.

In the North, hemp use increased, but not production, and so prices rose. In the South, excess cotton was sold overseas for money to help with the war effort. When the war was over, hemp had lost its hold to cotton. Wood was beginning to be used for paper, ships were being built of steel with steam engines and didn't need sails; steel cables replaced roping. Industry came and the age of hemp was over in the United States.[21]

Cannabis as Medicinal

By the middle of the 1800s, cannabis began to show up in American pharmacies. It was most often prescribed as a pain reliever and antibiotic. Doctors liked to prescribe it as a pain reliever, as the only other alternatives at the time were addic-

....

20. Deitch, *Hemp: American History Revisited*, 15.

21. Booth, *Cannabis: A History*, 45.

tive opiates, and they knew cannabis was not addictive. Read that again. In the 1800s, doctors knew opiates were addictive and cannabis was not. They knew cannabis was less expensive and didn't produce negative side effects like opiates did.[22] They knew this—over one hundred fifty years ago, they knew this, but today we are arguing about whether cannabis is better to give to patients or if opiates are. And then we wonder why there is an opiate addiction problem in our country. Maybe it's because our own government and doctors created one.

As the century wore on, cannabis was eventually approved to treat alcoholism, anthrax, anxiety, cholera, dysentery, epilepsy, migraines, neuralgia, opiate addiction, tetanus, typhus, and much more.[23] So again, we see cannabis was in good standing with the people and the medical field. People knew cannabis was helpful. At one point, it became the number four ingredient in medications in America. It had many uses and was quite versatile. While it was often in a tincture, pill forms were also used in pharmaceuticals. It's hard to believe it went from being so popular to outlawed. What was able to change the minds of Americans about such a helpful plant? Sadly, hate and greed were the two biggest contributors.

....

22. Booth, *Cannabis: A History*, 109, 113.
23. Booth, *Cannabis: A History*, 113–114.

Racial Intolerance Meets Federal Law

Several small steps eventually led to the complete ban of hemp and cannabis in America. These steps came from more than one direction at the same time.

Many Chinese people had come to participate in the California Gold Rush, and when they came, they brought with them opium habits. This scared white people who began associating Chinese people with opium.

While many white people did not know of the psychoactive effects of cannabis by the early 1900s, many African Americans did know because in Africa, cannabis was known as "dagga" and they were experienced with its use. Stolen and sold as slaves, they still had customs they brought with them and handed down to future generations. While cannabis (hemp) was still being grown for fibers, they were able to cultivate and dry the flowers for smoking.[24]

The use of cannabis in Mexico became prevalent as cannabis, which had once been cultivated, began growing in the wild, making it free. As more Mexican people emigrated to the United States, they brought their customs with them.

Since not too many white people smoked cannabis for recreational purposes, they were able to use it as an excuse to be against those who did. Between the influx of immigrants, the freeing of slaves, and the sudden growth in the use of drugs, fear and racism had begun to grow. Anything

....

24. Booth, *Cannabis: A History*, 155–156.

nonwhite people did was seen as un-American. This included the smoking of "marijuana." Part of the problem was critics didn't call it *cannabis* either. Cannabis was the helpful medicine in the pharmacy. The critics called it *marijuana* instead, and white people were fooled—they didn't understand the cannabis in the pharmacy was the same thing as the marijuana being smoked.

In 1906, the Pure Food and Drug Act required listing ingredients on medicines crossing state lines. This was a step forward in lumping cannabis in with more dangerous ingredients such as cocaine, morphine, and opium.

In 1914, El Paso passed a law banning marijuana after a fight broke out. The reason for the law wasn't so much about cannabis itself, as it was about controlling the Mexican population. Once neighboring towns saw how well it worked in controlling immigrants, they began incorporating the same type of laws. When marijuana came into town, people were arrested, fines were paid, people were jailed, and a free work force was created. In the same year, the Harrison Narcotics Act required record keeping of, and taxes to be paid on, purchases of narcotics. While cannabis was originally included in the first drafts of the Act, it was finally excluded due to how common of an ingredient it was. The states decided to take matters into their own hands, and by 1934, thirty-three states had banned cannabis other than as a medicine.[25]

....

25. Booth, *Cannabis: A History*, 161–162.

Throughout the country, white men began spreading the fear that people of color were out to corrupt white people with their usage of marijuana. The Mexican people in Texas, Sikhs and Punjabis in California, and Caribbean and West Indian immigrants in New Orleans were all targeted in different campaigns of hate and control. These people all had a history of cultural cannabis use, but instead of dropping the use when they came to America, they brought it with them, and white men especially saw this as a threat to their status quo. Louisiana cracked down so hard in 1926, the punishment for possession was six months in prison or a fine of $5,000.[26] In comparison, $5,000 in 1926 is equivalent to about $73,000 in 2020. By the 1930s, cannabis use had spread to most of the major United States cities, but still was used mainly by minorities. While the National Prohibition Act had started to clean up America, politicians (again, white men) saw the opportunity to go after what they saw as other vices—tobacco, jazz, and marijuana.

Greedy Men and a Conspiracy

Randolph Hearst was a rich man. He was also a greedy and unliked man who wanted to cut down a forest in Mexico for the wood to make paper for his newspaper. Hearst had a stake in paper being made from wood and didn't like the competition hemp provided either since hemp could produce four times the amount of paper as wood per acre.

....

26. Booth, *Cannabis: A History*, 165.

Long story short, Pancho Villa and his compatriots didn't like the idea of Hearst taking over the land and forest in Mexico, and they stopped it from happening. This incident eventually led to the Mexican Border Campaign and then the Mexican Revolution. In order to get public sentiment on his side, Hearst began a campaign of hate against Mexican immigrants by focusing on their cannabis use—only he didn't call it *cannabis*—he called it *marijuana*. His newspapers published sensationalized stories known as yellow journalism to garner readers. Many of these stories proclaimed the dangers of marijuana. What Hearst kept hidden was marijuana was really the same thing as the hemp and cannabis Americans had been using and growing for hundreds of years, even if those uses and demands had changed over the centuries.[27]

Though the use of hemp had been dying out, a new invention promised to revive the use of it. The decorticator made hemp easier to process with far less labor by being able to separate the fibers and seeds the same way the cotton gin had with cotton.[28]

Hearst had his interest in keeping the hemp industry down, but he wasn't the only one. There are different ways of making plastics. Plastics can be petroleum based (what most of us are used to) or hemp based (which, thanks to recent changes in laws, are finally making a comeback). The barons of the petroleum industry—the Mellon, DuPont,

....

27. Deitch, *Hemp: American History Revisited*, 88–89.

28. Deitch, *Hemp: American History Revisited*, 116.

and Rockefeller families—all had a huge stake in ensuring petroleum-based plastics were the wave of the future over hemp-based plastics. The four families stood to lose in the fuel, paper, and plastic industries if hemp replaced both wood and petroleum. As the largest donors, and therefore controllers, of the Republican party, they needed the laws to back them and their interests.[29]

While Andrew Mellon served as Secretary of the Treasury in June 1930, the Treasury Department created the Federal Bureau of Narcotics, and Mellon placed his nephew-in-law, Harry J. Anslinger, as the commissioner.[30] Political favors and nepotism were all they needed to complete their mission of destroying a competitive industry and therefore maintaining their hold and the status quo.

Once Anslinger realized he could get more money for the FBN if he had a new enemy on the forefront, he, too, picked up the battle against marijuana—and along with it, Black and Hispanic people. He won. By 1936, thirty-eight states listed marijuana on their list of most dangerous drugs. He himself wrote pamphlets claiming marijuana used by Black and Mexican people turned them into rapists and murderers—with the victims generally being white females. There was no evidence for this, of course, but it didn't matter. As Anslinger's

....

29. Deitch, *Hemp: American History Revisited*, 117.

30. Deitch, *Hemp: American History Revisited*, 119.

word spread, more people jumped on the bandwagon to ban a plant they really knew nothing about.[31]

Along with the bad press in the papers, several anti-marijuana movies were released. Marijuana soon became associated with violence and other crimes (theft, rape, murder). It was associated with sex and promiscuity. Use of marijuana at the time was not widespread to begin with, so those who feared it quickly outnumbered those who used it.

The Marijuana Tax Act

Anslinger was a master of propaganda. It may have taken him a while, but he eventually gained the support of the Treasury Department and the Marijuana (Marihuana) Tax Act of 1937 was passed. While marijuana was not made illegal, the act put an incredibly large tax on it and required an abundance of paperwork to register with the federal government if you were a manufacturer, importer, seller, or consumer. The act was designed to discourage anyone from wanting to have anything to do with marijuana. It discouraged them so much, extraordinarily little was ever collected in taxes.[32] The written act was not presented to the House Ways and Means Committee in advance of their session, so they would not be able to oppose it. Lies ruled, facts were ignored, and most importantly, the tie between marijuana and hemp and cannabis was completely hidden. Congress passed the act with no idea what they had just done, and what they had done was destroy

....

31. Booth, *Cannabis: A History*, 180–182.

32. Deitch, *Hemp: American History Revisited*, 146–147.

the entire hemp industry and contribute to another economic depression. Anslinger had done such a good job with his propaganda campaign, the members of Congress had no idea that marijuana was the same thing as the cannabis in the pharmacies and the hemp growing in the fields prized for its strong fiber. Anslinger's deceit destroyed not only industries, but it also destroyed people.

Although hemp wasn't as popular as it had once been, it was still being used in the United States for many different types of products. The Marijuana Tax Act immediately closed those businesses down, as the tax was extremely high and unaffordable.

Grow Hemp for Victory

Four years after Anslinger convinced Congress to wipe out the hemp industry, it suddenly became in demand again after Japan provoked the US into the war with the bombing of Pearl Harbor in December 1941. Hemp was needed so badly in the war effort, the government did a one-eighty on hemp and began the "Grow Hemp for Victory" campaign. Even children were encouraged to grow cannabis to help with the effort. Hemp was vital for naval supplies, and hemp seed oil worked as an airplane lubricant. When the war ended, so did the program. Fields of hemp were left unharvested and seeds spread on the wind. Hemp became a weed no one cared about.[33]

....

33. Booth, *Cannabis: A History*, 192–193.

Anslinger Doesn't Give Up

Anslinger held his position for over thirty years and spent a great deal of time battling against cannabis/hemp/marijuana. He blamed rising crime rates and Communism on marijuana. Ainslinger started the belief cannabis was a "gateway" drug and led to heroin use. In 1951, with the passage of the Boggs Act, he was able to go after users and focused on people in the entertainment industry. In 1956, the Narcotics Control Act passed Congress with help from Ainslinger. This act upped imprisonment to a five-year sentence for possession. In 1961, he convinced the United Nations to outlaw marijuana. With the election of President Kennedy, Anslinger saw the end of his career when forced into retirement. Kennedy was said to have smoked marijuana in the Oval Office himself, and so his views were at quite different odds from Anslinger. The damage Anslinger did, however, led to the incarceration of thousands and thousands of people, mainly men of color. It destroyed the hemp industry. Many people lost their livelihoods, and it was all based on lies. Worse yet, it set the tone on cannabis for decades to come.[34]

One War Sparks Another

By the time the '60s and '70s rolled along, the use of recreational cannabis had spread throughout the country. Music had been a counterpart to marijuana for years, starting with the birth of jazz in New Orleans. As musicians travelled, they

....

34. Deitch, *Hemp: American History Revisited*, 165–166.

spread their knowledge of marijuana with them. Thanks to Anslinger's and Hearst's campaigns, the name "marijuana" stuck. Much of the music and musicians of the '60s and '70s didn't hide their usage; instead, it was often celebrated, much to the dismay of more conservative voices.

At the same time this was happening in America, thousands of young American men were fighting thousands of miles away from home in the small country of Vietnam. Many of those young Americans took advantage of the easily available cannabis. It helped them to de-stress. When they came home, they continued to use it to help deal with the aftereffects of the war.

With the amount of rebellion happening on American soil with protests and demonstrations—often by people who used cannabis and were encouraged by liberal musicians—the government cracked down by stepping up the war on drugs. Conservatives raged a war against liberals for having different ideologies. Making cannabis illegal was a way to control the people who used it and lock them up and out of the way when they shared ideas different from the ones the powers that be held. For a country supposedly based on freedom, these types of laws have never made a ton of sense.[35]

In May 1969, the US Supreme Court in Leary v. United States, struck down the Marijuana Tax Act, saying it was unconstitutional. For thirty years, cannabis and hemp had

---

35. Deitch, *Hemp: American History Revisited*, 169–170.

been federally illegal; with the Supreme Court decision, it was once again federally legal, though many states still had laws against it.

While John F. Kennedy and Lyndon Johnson had been more focused on Vietnam than on worrying about the use of marijuana, Nixon saw it as an enemy to his political career. Woodstock had showed the country the propaganda against cannabis was nothing but lies. Thousands of people used it together in one location, and the problems supposedly associated with its use failed to appear. No murders. No fights. No crazed rapist rampages. Woodstock emphasized peace and love over hate and control. Nixon reacted with a crackdown in the form of Operation Intercept—a program where border agents searched every vehicle coming into the United States from Mexico specifically looking for cannabis. While the program only lasted three weeks and was expensive and a huge failure, it did make the transportation of cannabis into the country much more difficult. In 1970, Congress approved the Controlled Substances Act, which classified cannabis as a Schedule 1 substance, labeling it just as dangerous as heroin.[36] A Schedule 1 drug is considered to have no medical use. History tells us, though, this is not true of cannabis, as it had already been used for hundreds of years as an effective medicine.

....

36. Deitch, *Hemp: American History Revisited*, 180.

In 1973, the Commission on Marijuana and Drug Abuse suggested to Nixon that small amounts of cannabis be allowed for sale and use. Their study showed no one had ever died from cannabis use and there was literally no reason to consider it dangerous and illegal. While many people from all walks of life agreed, President Nixon did not, and so he rejected the recommendations of his own commission.[37]

It turns out several reports over the years all sided with cannabis not being a dangerous substance. These studies included the Indian Hemp Drugs Commission Report in 1894; the Panama Canal Zone Study, 1925; the LaGuardia Commission Report, 1944; the book *Licit and Illicit Drugs* published in 1972; Consumers Union follow-up to *Licit and Illicit Drugs*, 1975; the 1980 Drug Abuse Council's Report; and a 1982 study by the National Academy of Sciences.[38]

The stance President Ronald Reagan took on cannabis in the 1980s was downright ridiculous. He reinstated mandatory prison sentences and used the military to enforce drug laws. In less than twenty-five years, the percentage of people in federal jails for drug crimes went from sixteen to sixty-two. It was a great way for the government to seize the property of these "criminals." The power Reagan granted to law enforcement for property seizure was, in effect, another witch hunt on American soil. People went to jail for miniscule amounts

....

37. Booth, *Cannabis: A History*, 298.

38. Deitch, *Hemp: American History Revisited*, 184–185.

of a plant. People lost homes, cars, money, possessions—all because the government said no to a plant they knew was not harmful. It was far more about control than it ever was about health or safety. It should come as no surprise that those targeted the most were Black men. Drug tests for work became the norm. Reagan authorized the mass spraying of chemical herbicides in national forests to combat illegal grows, which, by the way, killed all kinds of other vegetation and couldn't have been too great for the animals or water supply either.[39]

In 1992, President George H. W. Bush ended the federal compassionate marijuana use program run by the National Institute of Drug Abuse. It had continually denied patients' applications anyway, but due to some lawsuits, the federal government still had to supply cannabis to around a dozen people. This cannabis is grown at a government-run research facility at the University of Mississippi, which has been studying cannabis for decades.[40] The government even holds patents on specific strains, while they continually enact laws to control certain segments of the population while ignoring their own evidence of the effects of cannabis.

For decades, the government used its power to control specific parts of the population by criminalizing a plant, which was not only safe but also beneficial to many people.

....

39. Booth, *Cannabis: A History*, 307–309.

40. Deitch, *Hemp: American History Revisited*, 210.

Money, greed, and dominance have been the main reasons for the illegalization of cannabis.

A Growing Interest

In 1989, the Business Alliance for Commerce in Hemp was formed. They found loopholes into importing hemp and started researching how hemp could be used. One of the member companies began importing hemp canvas from China. After Willie Nelson began promoting hemp, interest grew even more. In 1991, the American Hemp Council was formed. Within five years, three hundred businesses were manufacturing hemp products—but they could not grow the hemp themselves. It had to be imported because of the pesky Marijuana Tax Act of 1937. In 1999 in Hawaii, the federal government allowed hemp-growing for the first time in forty years.[41]

The more interest grew, the more uses for hemp people discovered—whether from other countries who weren't afraid of hemp the way Americans were or from research done here. Hemp is incredibly versatile and can be made into literally thousands and thousands of different types of products: from plastics, to building materials, fabric, toiletries, food, fuel, and many, many more. It has other benefits, since it grows much faster than trees; things like paper (including toilet paper and paper towels) can be grown with less environmental impact. Hemp can even be made into lumber. It is

....

41. Booth, *Cannabis: A History*, 342–343.

an easily renewable, quick-growing resource, and for years it remained illegal.

In the 2004 court case Hemp Industries Association v. DEA the Ninth Circuit Court sided with the HIA and permanently protected the sale of hemp body care and food products. Ten years later, President Barack Obama signed the Farm Bill into law, allowing for hemp farming pilot programs. The distinction between hemp and cannabis was legally defined as hemp contains less than 0.3 percent THC. The first attempt to fully legalize hemp came a year later in 2015. Unfortunately, it took another three years before legislation was passed in the Agriculture Improvement Act of 2018. This law finally removed hemp, its seeds, oils, etc., from the Controlled Substances Act. Unfortunately, cannabis remains on that list.

With the legalization of hemp, CBD has become abundantly available, and people can finally, legally, benefit from it. Research is being done by more than just government-run facilities, and new developments and products are constantly being discovered and created.

"Hemp," "cannabis," "marijuana"—all three name the same plant, but each have quite different connotations. Perhaps it is time we demand our government stop the lies and start demanding the cover-up be undone.

From being an important part of the beginning of the colonies and country to being banned to make the rich richer and the poor more controllable to being back on the rise again, hemp has had a roller coaster of a history in the United States.

CHAPTER 2

Science: The Magic of the Plant

In this chapter, we are going to learn about what CBD is and how—along with why—it works with our bodies (and the bodies of other animals too). While the last chapter was the history, this chapter is the science and magic, because when it comes right down to it, this science is pure magic. However, because there are entire books on the complicated science of cannabis, and we are constantly learning more every day, we are only going to cover the basics. The cannabis knowledge base is constantly growing, but there is some key information everyone using CBD or other cannabinoids should understand and have as a starting point. This chapter is going to cover many different aspects—from what cannabinoids are to finding a reputable supplier to dosing information, because these are all a part of the science and magic of CBD.

Cannabinoids

What are cannabinoids and what is CBD? Cannabis plants contain many different chemical compounds. These compounds are known as cannabinoids. One of these cannabinoids is cannabidiol, also known as CBD. Since this is a compound occurring naturally in the plant, it is a phytocannabinoid. CBD is only one of the many chemical compounds found in the cannabis plant. Over a hundred cannabinoids have been identified by researchers, and over another three hundred chemical compounds.

While CBD has become increasingly popular over the last several years, its use is by no means new, as we have seen. CBD has been in use for thousands of years, generally through smoking or in a tea-like beverage, or in later years, the medicinal cannabis tinctures and pills. Now that scientists know how to isolate CBD, we can use it in a form separate from the plant it comes from.

CBD—the compound—was not discovered until 1940. THC (tetrahydrocannabinol) was discovered twenty-four years later in 1964. THC is the cannabinoid that gives you the feel of a high. CBD does not have this same type of effect.

The Endocannabinoid System

Did you know your body contains an endocannabinoid system? Just like your circulatory system or digestive system, there is a system throughout your body that is designed to work specifically with cannabinoids. Cannabis produces compouds our bodies are biologically designed to use. This helps us see we need to work with nature and not against her. We are literally designed to be at our peak when we do.

The endocannabinoid system (ECS) is designed to help the body achieve and maintain homeostasis. It deals with energy, stress, and pleasure. When the body is balanced in these areas, health is at its peak.[42]

Our bodies produce endocannabinoids, neural chemicals in the nervous system that connect to several other bodily systems including the digestive, reproductive, and immune systems. The ECS then works with the phytocannabinoids in cannabis to produce results or a boost in those other systems. Similar to how your body's respiratory system works with air, your endocannabinoid works with cannabinoids.[43]

What this means is, the endocannabinoid system, which helps to keep our bodies in balance and therefore at their optimum functions, can be boosted with the phytocannabinoids found in cannabis plants to perform better, which then helps other bodily systems to perform better.

Part of the endocannabinoid system are what are called CB1 and CB2 receptors. Normally these receptors receive endocannabinoids produced by the neurons in our own bodies.

....

42. Eileen Konieczny, *Healing with CBD: How Cannabidiol Can Transform Your Health Without the High*, with Laura Wilson (Berkeley, CA: Ulysses Press, 2018), 47.

43. Leonard Leinow and Juliana Birnbaum, *CBD: A Patient's Guide to Medicinal Cannabis* (Berkeley, CA: North Atlantic Books, 2017), xxii.

These endocannabinoids are called N-arachidonoylethanolamine (AEA), also known as anandamide, and 2-arachidonoylglycerol (2-AG). But when we consume phytocannabinoids such as CBD or THC, these receptors are activated. Since our bodies only produce so many endocannabinoids at a time, we can use phytocannabinoids to flood our systems with the healing cannabinoids create. This is how we get the therapeutic benefits—by increasing our intake of cannabinoids over what our body already produces. New studies are showing a compromised endocannabinoid system—one deficient in either cannabinoid production or regulation—may be the cause of autoimmune disorders.[44] This would explain why cannabis is so effective in treating so many autoimmune conditions. CB1 and CB2 receptors are located throughout the many different systems of the body, with most CB1 receptors being in the brain and most CB2 receptors found in the immune system.[45]

As someone who used to be on massive painkillers along with several other medications for arthritis, fibromyalgia, and ankylosing spondylitis, I have been able to replace all of them, including a biologic injection, with nothing but good, old-fashioned cannabis. I spent thousands and thousands of dollars and decades of my life suffering when real

....

44. Toby K. Eisenstein and Joseph J. Meissler, "Effects of Cannabinoids on T-cell Function and Resistance to Infection," *Journal of Neuroimmune Pharmacol* 10 (2015): 204–216, https://doi.org/10.1007/s11481-015-9603-3.

45. Konieczny, *Healing with CBD*, 52–55.

relief could have been available to me years and years ago. Everyone should be allowed the health benefits of cannabis through CBD, THC, and other cannabinoids without it being a criminal act. The science doesn't change simply because the intent of the consumer may.

The Entourage Effect

CBD can obviously be used on its own, but it works best in conjunction with the other cannabinoids found in the cannabis plant. This is what is known as the entourage effect as discovered by Dr. Raphael Mechoulam in 1998.[46] What this means is CBD, THC, and all the other cannabinoids, along with terpenes, work best together. Each gives the others a boost or helping hand in different ways.

For example, when smoking a CBD strain of cannabis, you will get a decent entourage effect, as the flower bud you are smoking contains all the different chemical compounds and nothing has been isolated out of the flower. It is complete and whole as it is. Another way to obtain all the chemical compounds together is through what we call full-spectrum CBD. Full-spectrum products pull all the compounds from the plant and will include other phytocannabinoids, such as THC, but in order for it to be legal, the THC level must be below 0.3 percent terpenes, acids, and flavonoids.

....

46. Jamie Evans, *The Ultimate Guide to CBD: Explore the World of Cannabidiol* (Beverly, MA: Fair Winds Press, 2020), 15.

There are two issues with achieving the entourage effect. The first issue is the legality of THC. Since, as of this writing, cannabis is still federally illegal and not legal in all states, a full entourage effect itself is then illegal. Even though CBD can contain up to 0.3 percent THC, this is such a small amount, it is unable to produce a full effect. Does it help some? Yes. But more THC will allow the CBD and other cannabinoids to work better. The whole is better than the sum of its parts, but many people are being legally denied the whole.

The second issue is that some people do not like, nor want, the mind-altering effects of THC, or may not want them all the time, such as when driving or working. These problems make broad-spectrum CBD and CBD isolate good options in place of cannabis.

A broad-spectrum product has had the THC removed from it, but the other cannabinoids and terpenes remain. A CBD isolate is pure CBD—all other chemical compounds have been removed and the CBD is isolated, hence the name.

When I have a particularly painful day or get injured, I supplement my normal cannabis intake with extra doses of either full- or broad-spectrum CBD. Not only does this help control the pain, but CBD also helps counter the high of THC and creates more of an entourage effect, with the CBD giving a boost to the other cannabinoids and terpenes.

Terpenes

Terpenes are chemical compounds in plants and animals that act as cellular messengers. They are oils that have strong scents and flavors. There are many different terpenes, so we are going to limit our discussion down to the five most common to hemp/cannabis. Each of these terpenes have their own special magic to share with their user. Terpenes are what give cannabis its incredibly strong scents. It isn't often you will find a cannabis plant not highly fragrant no matter what its THC or CBD content is.

Pinene

If you have ever smelled a pine tree, you have smelled pinene. It is antiseptic, anti-inflammatory, an expectorant, and a bronchodilator (unless you happen to be allergic to it). Traditional Chinese Medicine says it fights against cancer. Pinene helps improve memory and concentration and counters THC's effects.

Linalool

Linalool is the floral scent in lavender. It is a sleep aid and helps to calm anxiety. It brings feelings of peace and relaxation. It activates immune cells and gives the immune system a boost. It is an anti-inflammatory and a weapon against Alzheimer's disease. It can help counteract anxiety caused by THC.

Beta-Caryophyllene

Beta-caryophyllene is a peppery scent. It is the only terpene known to work directly with the ECS, as it can bind with the CB2 receptor. It is an antioxidant, anti-inflammatory, and antinociceptive. It can be used to treat neuropathy and arthritic pain when combined with CBD.

Myrcene

Myrcene is the most common terpene in cannabis. It is what gives it the musky, dank, earthy smell. Myrcene is a sedative and allows CB1 receptors to hold on to more cannabinoids, which allows for THC to have a stronger effect or a stronger "high." It can treat insomnia and pain and is an analgesic, anti-inflammatory, and antibiotic.

Limonene

Limonene is the strong citrusy smell of lemons. It is energizing and uplifting along with being antifungal. It helps promote well-being, focus, and attention span. Smelling limonene will counteract the anxiety and high feeling of THC. In fact, inhaling the scent of lemon oil is a recommended way to combat a THC "overdose."[47]

Knowing the effects of different terpenes can help you choose strains or create custom products to work precisely in the way you need them. The whole is greater than the sum of the parts. Remember the entourage effect and how terpenes and cannabinoids join together to boost each other more.

....

47. Leinow and Birnbaum, *CBD: A Patient's Guide*, 29–34.

Characteristics and Benefits of CBD

While CBD is psychoactive, it is not intoxicating. There is a big difference between the two. THC gives you the intoxicating effect; CBD does not, but that does not mean it is not psychoactive. It's because it is psychoactive that it works to help heal certain ailments.

CBD is known for being a broad-range anti-inflammatory, which works in both the body and the brain by stimulating both CB1 and CB2 receptors and blocking the enzyme breakdown of anandamide in our systems. CBD prevents the reabsorption of adenosine, a neurotransmitter. This is how it can reduce both inflammation and anxiety.

CBD can bind with some non-cannabinoid receptors, resulting in many therapeutic benefits, including easing nausea and vomiting, eliminating seizures, and fighting tumors and cancer. It has antipsychotic, anti-inflammatory, antioxidant, antidepressant, and anti-anxiety properties.[48]

When you combine all these benefits together, it is easy to see how CBD can help bring a person into stronger, better, more stable health. It is easy to see how CBD suddenly became so popular. If it didn't work, the business would be failing, not growing exponentially.

Bioavailability

Bioavailability refers to how much and how fast a medicine is absorbed into the bloodstream. Depending on the way CBD

....
48. Konieczny, *Healing with CBD*, 90–91.

is used, it will affect its bioavailability. When CBD is taken orally, it must first be digested and go through the liver before it enters the bloodstream. This takes time and offers a lower bioavailability. THC, however, has a higher bioavailability than CBD when ingested and will produce stronger results.

Full-spectrum products have a higher bioavailability than do broad spectrum or isolates due to the entourage effect we discussed earlier. Studies have shown when it comes to CBD, edibles and pills have the lowest bioavailability levels. The highest rates come from smoking, vaping, sublinguals (under the tongue where it absorbs quickly), and suppositories. All these methods bypass the digestive system.[49]

CBD and Other Medications

CBD can affect other medications, so it is imperative to speak with your health professional before beginning any kind of a CBD supplement. This includes any forms taken internally, whether in a beverage, food, smoking, vaping, pills—anything consumed. It is possible to cause liver damage if some medications are combined with CBD, so we cannot stress enough the importance of being sure it will not have any harmful interactions before using. People want to be able to use CBD to feel better, not worse, so always make sure to double-check with your physician first.

....

49. Evans, *The Ultimate Guide to CBD*, 23.

Acids and Decarboxylation

Some products, you will find, contain information about things such as CBDA or THCA. These are slightly different than CBD and THC as they are the cannabinoid with an acid molecule attached. This secondary metabolite helps the plant fight off pests. With a little bit of magical science, we apply heat to the acid molecules, the acid burns off, and we are left with the cannabinoid. Decarboxylation is the process in which we apply the heat to convert those acids. This becomes important to know if you ever want to use your own flower to make products such as oils, butters, or tinctures and if you plan on doing any cooking with your flower. The total values are usually listed on packaging when you purchase flower products, but if you grow your own, you would have to get testing done on your flower to find out what the levels are, and this can be costly.

If your strain is already low in CBDA and high in CBD, you don't have to worry about it. However, say you buy some flower and it says it is 5 percent CBD and 10 percent CBDA. If you are smoking the flower, you are fine, nothing to worry about. But if you wanted to jar-infuse some alcohol, not decarbing the flower first isn't going to give you very strong CBD. You have to burn off that acid molecule, converting it all to CBD, which would then give you 15 percent CBD.

There are different ways to decarboxylate. When you smoke flower, the igniting of the flower does the job. When you want to use flower to infuse other products, you must first decarboxylate it in order to convert all the acid molecules for the fullest effect.

There are decarboxylators available for purchase for home use. They are not terribly expensive and are easy to use—you simply pour your flower into the container, pop the lid on, plug it in, and press a button. The decarboxylator heats up and bakes the acids out for you. It shuts off automatically.

You can use a slow cooker to decarb your flower. First, place your ground flower into a mason jar and seal tight. Fill a slow cooker at least halfway full of water. Place the jar into the water and set your slow cooker to high for four hours. After two hours, gently shake the jar to redistribute the flower. When the four hours is done, carefully remove the jar from the water and allow it to cool completely before opening. This will help keep the smell down. If you don't want the smell inside, be sure to open the jar outside to let it air for a moment.

You can also decarb your flower in your oven. This method does make the entire house smell of flower though, so be forewarned. Grind your buds and spread them out on a cookie sheet. Bake in an oven preheated to 225°F for 60 minutes.

No matter which method you use, always allow the flower to cool and then store it in an airtight jar. The magic has been performed, and the flower is ready to be used in future concoctions.

Science Is Your Friend

What if you don't want to make your own products from flower? Not a problem; there are many products on the market these days—everything from beverages to makeup to concentrated oils and transdermal patches. In fact, there is so much, it can be downright confusing to know what you are really getting.

Unfortunately, with any new booming market, fraud is going to find its way in. This is the downside of lack of oversight. Several TV news shows (and since then other research studies) have shown us what's inside the bottle may not always be what is advertised on the outside.[50] Sadly, there are many unreputable companies and dealers selling CBD products with absolutely no CBD in them.

But don't worry; once again, it is science to the rescue. The easiest way to find out if a company is reputable is to ask for information. If they can't, or won't, answer your questions, feel free to move on to another vendor. Ask where they source their hemp from. Is it organic? Research the company online. Do they do third-party testing? Are those tests results available to you? Any company not willing to give you this information is not worth working with. Use the available

....

50. Maria Cohut, "FDA Report Evaluates CBD Product Labeling Accuracy," Medical News Today, Healthline Media, October 29, 2020, https://www.medicalnewstoday.com/articles/fda-report-evaluates -cbd-product-labeling-accuracy#CBD-content-mislabeled,-THC-not -specified.

science to find reputable companies and products, because reputable companies will be more than happy to share the science with you.

When buying hemp products, the things you want to know include cannabinoid concentrations, all active ingredients, all inactive ingredients, brand name, location of where it was manufactured, and contact information for the company. Products with more than 0.3 percent THC may contain information about the type of cannabis used such as sativa/indica/hybrid, the name of the cultivar, and the types of terpenes it contains.

You may see on these hemp products that they do contain 0.3 percent THC. Yes, some hemp products do contain THC—remember, this is how the US government defines what is hemp and what is cannabis, so it may legally contain up to 0.3 percent THC and still be considered hemp. Do not worry; if you do not want to feel a high, you won't. There is nowhere near enough THC in these products to give you a high. That is why this level of THC is legal. It will not show up on a drug test. These are common misconceptions.

How Do They Get the CBD Out of the Plant?

Different types of hemp/cannabis are grown for CBD. Industrial hemp is low in CBD and is used for fibers and fuel. Drug hemp contains higher concentrations of CBD. Cannabis grown and sold for medical and recreational uses can be grown with different levels of CBD and THC.

If you are not using flower, your other option is a CBD concentrate after the CBD is extracted from the plant. There are many different extraction methods, some of which can be done at home. Others require special equipment and chemicals. The more the concentrate is processed, the more possibility of contaminants being introduced to the product. This, again, makes the science and third-party testing an important aspect of choosing which products to use.

The two main ways concentrates are extracted from the plant material are through either mechanical or chemical extraction.

We will start with chemical extraction, and you can probably already figure out the cons simply from the name of the process. Unfortunately, chemical extraction uses chemicals that may end up in the concentrate, which then end up in you. Ethanol, butane, CO_2, glycerin, and alcohol are all chemicals used to strip the compounds from the plant material.

Mechanically extracted concentrates can be made from techniques using sifters, heat, pressure, and even water. This will produce products such as hash, kief, and rosin.[51]

It all comes down to personal preference and how you feel about the process and possibilities of chemical contamination. It's another reason why third-party testing is so important. Companies that do not want third-party testing do not want it because they know what the testing will show.

....

51. Konieczny, *Healing with CBD*, 203–211.

I cannot stress enough the importance of being sure you can access data analysis regarding what you use.

Product Variety

There are so many CBD products on the market today; you can find many items you may want premade with it. But again, this doesn't mean you will have the best information on the actual CBD content. It takes research on the companies and their products to ensure you are getting what you are paying for. If you plan to use a lot of CBD products, it can become quite time consuming to be sure you aren't being scammed. While there are many great companies out there, there are unfortunately plenty of scammers too. Doing the research is worth the time to ensure you are getting a pure, quality product.

Remember the vape scare of 2019? All kinds of people ended up sick; some even died from illegal vaping products tainted with vitamin E oil. It is extremely important to verify your products are safe. At best, unsafe products do nothing, but they can do serious harm.

There are plenty of good, reliable, science-driven companies out there that have excellent, safe products, so don't be scared off; just be prepared to do your research to find who is worthy of your trust. Check with your friends and family. Look into references.

The other option is to find a good CBD supplier (like CryBaby CBD) and use those ingredients to make your own food, health, and beauty products yourself. This makes it easier to customize it to your needs for maximum benefits and results.

Companies like Cheryl's have done a lot of the research for you. Wanting to provide a high-quality product that works means she has already investigated and researched different growers and suppliers until she found the one she was not only willing to work with, but to bet her own reputation on. Not only does Cheryl run her own CBD business, but she is also her own client and uses the same products she recommends.

What you need is going to depend on what your purpose is. If you want to use CBD as a food additive or in health and beauty products such as lotions, soaps, or massage oil, concentrated CBD oil is the way to go. With capsules, lozenges, gummies, sprays, and oils, there are many ways to take CBD simply as a supplement too.

Later, we will go over different ways to add CBD into your life and guide you through several recipes to do so.

Dosing

When it comes to CBD, there are no standard dosing recommendations, so people aren't sure where to begin. There is almost too much information available for people to try to consume and decide what is best for them. When it comes right down to it, the only way to find out what works best for you is through trial and error.

Your beginning point depends on two key factors: what do you want to get out of the CBD (why are you taking it) and to start with a low dose.

First, let's talk about why you are wanting to use CBD. Are you looking for a daily supplement to boost your immune system? Do you suffer from chronic pain? Do you only want to use it occasionally as a natural pain reliever? There are many reasons people choose to take CBD. I take smaller doses throughout the day to help me deal with my daily pain along with the THC-filled cannabis I consume. This gets me through normal days. When I have a flare of one of my auto-immune disorders, I have to increase my intake of both THC and CBD for several days at a time. When I hurt myself, I need a large dose or several large doses to deal with the pain until it becomes more bearable and manageable with smaller doses. You may find you need and want different doses as I do, and this brings us to our second key point.

You should always begin with a low dose. You want to keep your body happy with the lowest doses possible. The reason behind this is … science! Using my case as an example, if my body was used to me taking a high dose daily, what happens when I have a flare? I would have to take an even higher dose to get my flare managed.

Since I have switched to treating myself with cannabis and CBD, I have had far fewer flares than when I was being highly medicated. I can physically do things I wasn't able to do when I was under the care of a rheumatologist and getting weekly injections of a chemotherapy drug that was supposed to stop and reverse the damage already done to my back, knees, and hips. It didn't. But it did make me ill for the several years I was on it, and I eventually ended up needing a walker to get around. I haven't needed a walker for years now, and I hope I won't need one again for decades to come.

Taking CBD for anxiety or to calm nerves is another reason to keep your dose low. If needed at some point, you can increase your dosage for stronger results. When your body and mind become used to one dose on a daily level, you need a higher dose for those little surprises life brings us.

When you first begin dosing, I cannot stress enough the importance of keeping a dosage journal. Document when you take your dose, how you take your dose, and what exactly the dose is. When do you start feeling any effects? Do you feel any effects? Remember, you might not for a while, or you may feel something really fast. How long do the effects last? Finding your dose requires a lot of listening to your body and checking for what may be slight changes at first.

Start your dosing low, wait, and see what you notice. If you are wanting a daily supplement just for a boost, you can start with a low-dose capsule—for example, 15 mg or 30 mg.

If you are looking to deal with anxiety, you can start with 15 mg several times a day (this is microdosing—we will discuss this more soon) and see if you notice any changes after a week. If you don't, go ahead and increase your dosage for another week, again looking for and observing any differences. Take notice of when you do begin feeling different. Use that dosage journal I recommended! There are plenty of dosage ranges available, so finding what works for you may happen quick, or it may take a while. Some pains and anxiety may show quick relief; they might not. I know, how aggravating. It is the downside, but it's a downside for a good reason. Every person's body is unique, and every person's body will react slightly different to CBD. We know what it does, but how much it takes for each person is not set in stone. It takes trial and error to find the right dosages for each person, but this also means it is customizable to you and your needs.

If you are looking to control chronic pain and inflammation, you may want to start off at a slightly higher strength and follow the same patterns. I don't know too many people who would get pain relief from a dose as low as 15 mg, but I'm not going to say it's not possible; maybe it is. What is important is whatever dose you start with, you pay attention to how you feel after taking it. One of the extra benefits of working with CBD, THC, or both is the connection it creates between you and your own body by paying extra-special attention to how it feels. Really paying attention. Not ignoring it, not a quick scan, but the way you learn to spend time inside your own body and connect with it. We will go over some meditations later to help you learn how to do this. I found muscles I didn't have any clue I had!

Cheryl's client Katie said, "After only a month I saw definite improvement to my aches and pains. I also feel a bit calmer." All it takes is finding what works best for you and understanding it isn't an overnight process to find your best zen.

As you learn more about your body and how CBD works with it, you will soon learn what dosages you need to maintain your own optimum health. Later, in "The Spirit" chapter, we will go over some meditations to help you learn how to check in with your body and see how it is doing on a regular basis.

CHAPTER 3

Pills, Potions, and Products: Finding What's Right for You

Before we dive into recipes and showing you how to incorporate CBD into your life, you need to think about what you are looking for in your CBD use. Your needs will help determine what types of products you want to use. There are five popular ways to administer CBD, those being: tincture (orally under tongue, sublingual), oral ingestion (capsules, sprays, edibles, concentrated oils), inhalation (vaped, smoked, dabbed), topical (on skin: lotions, creams, oils, beauty care products), and transdermal (patch on skin).

Types of CBD products

Let's talk about the different forms in which CBD can be used along with the pros and cons of each.

Flower

Flower or "bud" is the raw (dried) buds of the plant. This dried plant material may be smoked, vaporized, cooked, or infused into oils, butters, or tinctures.

Average time of onset for effects is 5–30 minutes after consumption. The average duration of feeling the active effects is 2–6 hours, though for some people, the effects may last up to 24 hours.

* *Pros:* Flower contains the most active chemical ingredients and has the highest concentrations of cannabinoids. It has the best use of the entourage effect, making it highly effective. It's the least processed—simply being grown and dried.

* *Cons:* Flower may contain higher percentages of THC unless it has been specifically grown and tested for less than 0.3 percent THC. If you grow your own, it will be impossible to know your THC levels without testing. Flower is still not yet legal everywhere due to the possible higher THC level. Legality issues and your own outlook on THC may lead to marks in the cons column.

Vapor Cartridges

Vape cartridges are extracted CBD oil. Remember from the science chapter, there are different ways of extracting the oils, which may include chemical solvents. Be sure to read labels, and if information is not provided, don't buy!

The average onset time is 5–30 minutes after consumption. The average duration of feeling the active effects is 2–6 hours and may last up to 24 hours. Vapor cartridges are inhaled.

* *Pros:* Vapes have a fast onset as the CBD molecules are sent to the lungs and absorbed almost immediately into the bloodstream. Vapes are generally good for quick relief of anxiety and chronic pain. They are helpful in treating sleep disorders and some forms of epilepsy. Vapes are discreet and have less odor than smoking.

* *Cons:* Safety issues with additives and metal contaminants. Be sure it comes from a reliable supplier, has a published ingredient list, has been batch tested by a third-party tester, and contains no additives or artificial flavorings.

Tinctures

Tinctures can be made with vegetable glycerin or a high-proof alcohol.

The average onset time is up to 2 hours, and the average duration of feeling the active effects is 12–24 hours. Tinctures be taken sublingually, orally, or applied topically.

* *Pros:* Tinctures are easy to use and amazingly fast acting when taken sublingually.

* *Cons:* Orally, tinctures take longer to take effect and have less bioavailability after digestion and passing through the liver to reach the bloodstream.

Oral Methods

Oral methods include foods, beverages, capsules, oils, and some tinctures. When taken orally, CBD enters the bloodstream through the digestive system instead of through the lungs, causing onset to be delayed up to 2 hours. Active effects may be felt for 12–24 hours.

* *Pros:* The doses are easy to take and have a long sustainability.
* *Cons:* Some methods do not taste great, and orally has a long activation time with less bioavailability.

Topicals

Topicals include balms, creams, lotions, massage oils, and cosmetic products. The onset for active effects can take 30 minutes to 2 hours. Those effects may last 1–6 hours. These types of products are used by applying them to skin or, as with some products such as shampoos or conditioners, to the hair. There are now a wide variety of CBD cosmetic products available including skin care, hair care, facial care, and deodorant.

* *Pros:* CBD topicals can provide pain relief without ingestion, making these products good for inflammation or joint conditions.
* *Cons:* Topicals only work on a skin-deep level; lotions and oils only allow a shallow penetration through the skin. For issues with inflammation and joint conditions, a topical works best when combined with an internal consumption method.

Transdermal Patch

Transdermal patches are filled with CBD that is absorbed through the skin into the bloodstream. They come in specific doses and can be worn for several days depending on the manufacturers' guidelines.

- ⋆ *Pros:* Transdermal patches are easy to use and to measure and control dosages.
- ⋆ *Cons:* They can take several hours to take effect, and it can take a while to find a dose that works well. Some people have allergic reactions to the adhesives.

Microdosing

How should you incorporate CBD into your life? Can you just take supplements? Yes, you can. But you can do so much more. Taking supplements is one thing, and those are great for when you have a flare and need an extra boost or a sudden larger dose for additional pain relief, but it is so boring. And honestly, the oils by themselves don't taste good. And you know what happens when you expect yourself to squirt a nasty-tasting oil into your mouth several times a day? You don't do it.

There are many ways you can incorporate CBD into your life that do not taste nasty. By being able to take your CBD in an enjoyable way, you will continue to take it—making those times when you need an extra boost or when you have a flare happen less often by bringing your body into a more perfect homeostatic balance through microdosing.

We touched on dosing a little bit before and how every person is different, making it difficult to find the dose you need. Microdosing is an extremely popular way to dose. Instead of taking one large dose in the morning or at night, microdosing is when you dose a little bit frequently throughout the day. This helps keep you at an even balance, with more CBD being activated as CBD from a previous consumption is wearing off. It's sort of like keeping a bucket with a small hole in the bottom filled. Keep adding slowly, and even though it's leaking, the bucket never empties. Microdosing works on a similar basis and keeps your body "filled" with CBD. This brings your body into a more balanced homeostasis. Achieving and maintaining a balanced state for your body can be life changing.

The difference for me has been astronomical. At one point in my life, I was basically living in a constant flare of all my several autoimmune disorders. The pain existed 90–95 percent of the time. The medications had uncomfortable side effects like water retention, massive drowsiness, weight gain, and memory loss, and they didn't take away the pain. I had to sleep in a recliner, not in a bed, as my back couldn't be straightened out due to spinal fusions from ankylosing spondylitis. I was severely hunched over and used a walker to get around. I had dozens of injections in my spine, sacroiliac joints, both my hips, a shoulder, and a knee. The medications made me feel like I was living in a haze. I have plenty of lost time from those days wiped from my memory due to the massive amounts of opiates I was being told to take by my doctor. My life was miserable. Once I made the decision I was done with the opiate medications, my life began a new path I never expected. I detoxed on my own. (Don't do that if you are on opiates and want to stop. It's dangerous.) I didn't know the danger at the time, nor did I know at the time my body had become completely addicted to them. This was several years before the words "opiate crisis" were ever uttered. I was terribly sick for about three weeks and at the time had no idea why. Now I know it was because my body was going through detox.

I had started acupuncture before my cold turkey opiate quit, and I believe it helped me get through it, though I don't know for sure. I had not yet started using cannabis to treat pain. I just knew what I had been doing for over a decade wasn't working, and I was tired of hearing the same old thing from the doctors telling me the things that weren't working should. They didn't work. I was tired of the way they made me feel. I was tired of the outrageous amounts of money I was spending to have such a lousy life. I was paying hundreds of dollars a month in medical and prescription costs after my insurance coverage. It was outrageous to spend so much money to not only still be in pain, but to make myself miserable in other ways besides!

Once I got off the opiates, my body started changing immediately. With acupuncture I was able to control most of my normal, daily pain, and I was far more coherent. I was living my life again. Then the breast cancer hit. Knowing I was not about to go back through all the opiate crud again, I opted for cannabis for pain and have been using both cannabis and CBD ever since. In non-COVID times, I maintained a few tune-up visits a year with my acupuncturists. My life is easily a thousand times better than what it was. For starters, I now have an actual life I can fully participate in and actually remember.

Anxiety, Pain, and Depression

I have been writing this book throughout the COVID-19 pandemic—an event that brought with it an abundance of anxiety and depression for millions of people who did not already suffer from these conditions. Hopefully, this new awareness of the staggering numbers of people who suffer from anxiety, pain, and depression begins the process of real changes, such as access to health care—including mental health care—for all. Remember, CBD is not a replacement for professional medical help. It's in addition to it.

Anxiety, pain, and depression can hit separately, in twos, or all at once. Having anxiety and depression leads to physical pain. Physical pain can lead to depression and anxiety. The three of them are often so intertwined, it's hard for the patient to even tell them apart.

CBD can not only help you separate those feelings—drawing the line between them—it can help you defeat them. Once you can focus on yourself and how you are feeling, it makes feeling better all the easier. Dealing with these three issues is where CBD does some of its best work.

Cheryl's client Whitney stated she began using CBD because "I've had severe anxiety for a few years now, and with COVID and teaching from home, anxiety attacks have been a daily occurrence. I asked around, and my friend let me try some of her CryBaby CBD oil. I went a week and a half without an anxiety attack... I ordered my own bottle of CBD oil and gummies."

Many people can eventually adjust or eliminate pharmaceuticals when they begin using CBD (again, though, with a doctor's guidance). Cheryl's client Joel said, "I have been taking CBD for quite a while now and I have found a good dosage that works for me. It's with great excitement that I can say I have (with a doctor's help) stopped taking my anxiety medication for weeks now! I can feel even more of the effects since I have been off prescription medication."

So, what can CBD do for you?

Cheryl's client Mary shows how CBD can have different uses. She said, "Hemp oil allows me to take on daily stress calmly and helps me to sleep deeper, waking refreshed. I began to also use the CBD hemp oil topically on my face twice a day. My sixty-four-year-old face loves it. After three weeks, I see clearer skin, wrinkles are receding, and my huge pores on my nose have shrunk to the point they are no longer visible. It is the best ever."

Client Jenni said, "I work out every day and this (CBD balm) soothes my achy muscles. I get it for my mother-in-law too. She has constant pain in her hip. She's been to doctors and physical therapy, and this is the only thing that gives her relief."

And because we've all been there too, Cheryl's client Kelly said, "I was skeptical of the whole CBD thing because it's so trendy right now … but tried it on myself. It's amazing."

Let's go over what a day in the life could look like with different options for incorporating CBD Again, it really depends on what you are looking for CBD to do for you, but I think this following example will give you plenty of ideas for where to start your own CBD regimen.

A Day in the Life

When you wake up in the morning, do you go straight for the coffee pot? CBD-infused coffee can help you start off your day feeling refreshed and focused, even if the coffee is decaffeinated. Tea drinker? You are covered too, either with coffee or tea products you buy already infused or ones you mix up yourself.

Time to brush your teeth and shower. CBD toothpaste is great for inflamed gums because it acts as a topical to help ease inflammation, it keeps healthy teeth healthy, and it will help absorb some of the CBD into your system. Sensitive teeth or gum pain? CBD can help numb both those pains. You can finish off with a CBD mouthwash to ensure you get in between teeth to tighter problem areas. Shampoo, conditioner, and soap are all available or can be homemade with CBD, which helps revitalize both hair and skin, keeping them supple while avoiding dryness. CBD in facial cleansers can help treat acne. Shave creams, body lotions, and face creams are all topical products that can be CBD infused to help with several different skin issues.

Breakfast, the most important meal of the day. Imagine a customized smoothie to help meet whatever your needs are. Customized, you ask? But how? This is where it starts to get fun. The terpenes found in cannabis species are found in many other foods, so you can look for foods rich in the terpenes you want to accentuate to combine with CBD, enhancing the—you guessed it—entourage effect! Voilà! Magic!

Throughout the day, there are several different ways you can microdose, vaping being an extremely popular one. At this point, it's important to point out the methods of consumption so far in this day have been through ingestion or contact (on the skin, hair, gums), which in most cases takes longer to take effect and does have lower bioavailability. This means even though we have consumed a bit of CBD, our bodies are not getting the full effect. Personally, the first thing I do in the morning after waking up and telling Alexa to snooze my alarm is to use my vape sitting on the night-stand next to my bed. As we learned earlier, using a vape has high bioavailability, as the CBD is absorbed through the lungs directly to the bloodstream. This gives me a jump start for the day while I snooze for a few more minutes and let my body begin to wake up. With my autoimmune disorders, getting out of bed in the morning is difficult, as my joints have had time to stiffen up from remaining stationary overnight. My first vaped dose in the morning is often the reason I can get out of bed at all! Sometimes I need a second dose when getting out of bed, sometimes not; it depends on things like the weather, what I did the day before, and even if I drank enough water.

Other ways to microdose throughout the day instead of vaping can include dosing with oils, CBD drinks, CBD gummies, or other snacks. Both your lunch and dinner can be infused with CBD in different ways.

Ready to relax after a long day of work? Unwind in a CBD bath to help ease physical pains and coax an overactive mind to unwind. Maybe have a CBD-infused cup of tea or night cap before bed.

Using CBD this way ensures you keep your levels up so you stay balanced throughout the day. This allows for maximum effect and maximum healing. Adding CBD into your life is more than just adding in a supplement. It's adopting a new way to do things to achieve maximum results and help your body achieve its best homeostasis levels to ensure proper function and healing take place. CBD and other cannabinoids act as a fuel to the endocannabinoid system. They can keep it running and producing all the goodness our bodies need.

Often, when I talk to people and they tell me neither CBD nor THC worked for them, I ask them about how they used it. Most often, they try it a couple times, usually with no guidance, and either have no reaction or a negative one (more common with THC). The problem with this is, unbeknownst to them, they weren't using it correctly to achieve the desired results. This sets them up for failure right off the bat. This is why education on how to use cannabinoids is so essential. When you learn to go slow and low and really connect with and listen to your body and build yourself up to what you need in a responsible manner, a whole new world opens to you. Trying once or twice honestly isn't doing it right. I hope you will spread this knowledge when you run into doubters—and you *will* run into doubters—people who do not understand the science and will tell you hemp/cannabis is not a miracle plant. But remember earlier? We already said it's not a miracle plant, but it is a magical one, backed up with scientific data showing it is designed to work with our bodies to help us heal.

CHAPTER 4

Starting from Scratch: Working with CBD Flower

Working with flower instead of buying concentrated oils or other premade products is often more economical, especially if you are growing your own plants to harvest. It is more work, obviously, but you then know precisely what soil, water, and fertalizers go into your own plants and final products. When you start off with flower, you can infuse it into different base products. These base ingredients can then be used in recipes as you normally would. You can put CBD butter on your toast every morning, or you can use it to bake CBD cookies. You can use CBD jojoba oil in a variety of massage, facial, and hair oils. You can use infused simple syrup to serve CBD cocktails to your friends. You can drink your tea sweetened with CBD honey. There are a variety of ways CBD can be used in your daily life, and these base ingredients are one key way of getting there.

CBD flower is easily available since it has federal legal status; it can be shipped through the mail, cross state lines, or be sold in stores. It is relatively inexpensive in flower form, making it a cost-effective alternative to CBD oils. Working with CBD flower also gives you the option of saving plant material after infusions to reuse in other ways, giving you even more for your money.

Earlier in this book, we talked about decarboxylation. If you are going to use flower as an ingredient, or to make other ingredients, you must first decarboxylate it with one of the methods we described before. After it is decarboxylated, it is ready to be made into an infusion or even used in its flower form as an ingredient. For the most part, you will want to use flower for infusions or for smoking. The main infusions you use will be made with butters, oils, and tinctures.

Remember, one of the benefits of working directly with flower is the entourage effect. It has the complete spectrum of cannabinoids (which may include THC, so know what you are working with), terpenes, and other chemical constituents that enable CBD to work better.

There are different methods available to infuse products with flower. The easiest of these methods is to use a machine specially designed to do it. The MagicalButter machine has been the best invention for people who want to produce their own infusions at home. It literally requires pouring in the ingredients, pressing some buttons, and then straining the bulk material out when the cycle completes. All you need to do is read what settings to use for different materials and then select the proper ones on the device. The Magical-Butter machine is available for less than $250. While it is not a necessity, it is a time-saver, and it produces higher-quality infusions than other at-home techniques, which in turn can save money and eventually pay for the machine.

Making your own concoctions means having some way to safely store them after they are made. Mason jars are your friends. They are great for holding buds, butters, honey, and both cooking and cosmetic oils. You will also need amber bottles with dropper tops. These come in an assortment of sizes, and you may want to stock up on several of each. They are perfect for simple syrup, alcohol infusions, and your final oil blends. Of course, you can get as fancy as you want with different jars and bottles—just ensure they seal airtight. It's best to keep your products out of direct sunlight. A dark cupboard shelf is an ideal spot to store your products.

Infused Butter (or Ghee)

Think of all the recipes you already use butter in. This is an easy way to add CBD into your normal routine by simply substituting regular butter or ghee with an infused version. Remember, the goal is to keep CBD coming into the body regularly to keep it at optimum levels. Infused butter is just one of the little ways it can become a part of your normal daily routine. This will work with cooking oils too.

Whichever you prefer is quite up to you. Ghee has a higher fat content level, which allows it to absorb more cannabinoids than regular butter does. It has a richer, more "buttery" taste than butter. It is butter intensified.

Remember, the flower and terpenes are going to change the taste. The butter will not taste quite like butter. If you don't like the taste, there are ways to help cover up some of it to make it more palatable. You can eliminate some odd tastes by checking out what type of terpenes are dominant in the strains available to you. If you don't want a piney taste, stay away from ones with pinene. Limonene strains will have a hint of a citrusy taste, which can be paired nicely with other herbs to change up the flavor. For example, buttering a piece of bread with infused butter is one way to eat it. Mixing the same butter with a little garlic salt before spreading it on the bread will alter the taste greatly. The key is to experiment. Mix up a batch of butter and try it out with different herbs and spices. Try it in different recipes. Increasing spices, herbs, and other flavorings helps to cover and counteract the tastes brought out from the flower in the infusion process.

If you do not have a MagicalButter machine, there are two other ways to infuse butter or ghee: the slow cooker method and the stove top method. The process is the same for both. The amount of flower you use is up to you, but you should use it in the recommended range given. The more you use, the stronger your final product will be, but the more expensive it will be too.

❉ *Flower-Infused Butter (Slow Cooker Method)*

Ingredients

- ⋆ ¼–½ cup of water (for 7 grams, use ¼; if you use the full 14 grams, go up to ½ cup)

- ⋆ 1 cup of butter or ghee

- ⋆ 7–14 grams ground decarboxylated flower

Utensils

- ⋆ Slow cooker

- ⋆ Wooden spoon

- ⋆ Spatula

- ⋆ Cheesecloth

- ⋆ Glass mason jar with lid

- ⋆ Spouted measuring cup

Pour the water into the slow cooker and add the butter or ghee. Set temperature to low (190°F). After the butter melts, add the flower and stir well with a wooden spoon and using a spatula to scrape down the sides. Allow to cook for 4 hours, scraping the sides and stirring every half an hour.

Place cheesecloth over the mason jar loosely and hold in place with the ring (not the lid, just the ring). Be sure to allow the cheesecloth to hang loosely inside. I kind of punch it down with my fist before tightening the ring so it creates a cavity to fill with the plant material. Using a spouted measuring cup, scoop the mixture out of the slow cooker and into the mason jar where the cheesecloth catches all the plant material. When you get to the bottom, you can tip the slow cooker to scrape and pour out the rest.

Allow the material to drip for a while. I prefer to squeeze mine out, but some people do not, as this runs the risk of allowing plant material to escape the cheesecloth into your butter. It's entirely up to you, but it is more economically sound to give it a squeeze. Store the butter in the refrigerator; when the butter hardens, any leftover water will separate, and you can remove it.

✿ Flower-Infused Butter (Stove Top Method)

Ingredients

* 1–2 cups of water (for 7 grams, use 1 cup; if you use the full 14 grams, go up to 2 cups)

* 1 cup of butter or ghee

* 7–14 grams ground decarboxylated flower

Utensils

* Small saucepan

* Wooden spoon

* Spatula

* Candy thermometer

* Cheesecloth

* Glass mason jar with lid

Place the small saucepan on the stove on low heat. Add the water and bring it to a simmer, then add the butter or ghee and allow it to melt. The water keeps the butter from burning, and more water may need to be added throughout the process. Add in the ground flower and stir gently with the wooden spoon, ensuring it is all covered and mixed in evenly. Keep the mixture simmering between 150° and 160°F. Do not let it boil. If the water evaporates, add more. Be sure to check on it and stir it every 15 minutes for 2–3 hours. Be sure to consistently scrape down the sides, as the plant material may stick. The longer you let it simmer, the more potent your butter will be.

Place cheesecloth over the mason jar loosely and hold in place with the ring (not the lid, just the ring). Be sure to allow the cheesecloth to hang loosely inside by pushing it down before tightening the ring so it creates a cavity to fill with the plant material. Carefully pour the saucepan contents into the mason jar, with the cheesecloth catching all the plant material.

Allow the material to drip for a while or squeeze out. Store the butter in the refrigerator; when the butter hardens, any leftover water will separate, and you can remove it.

Flower-Infused Oil

There are two different types of oils you are going to want to infuse: the kind you cook with and the kind you don't. What types of oils do you generally use when cooking? For baking I use vegetable oil, but for cooking I use either olive oil or occasionally coconut oil. For massage and cosmetic purposes, I use coconut and jojoba, so when I infuse oils, I do all four of them: coconut, jojoba, olive, and vegetable.

It can be expensive to do them all at once, so start with what you use the most and add more varieties when you can. Coconut is a great oil to work with since it can be used for both cooking and cosmetic purposes. Jojoba is preferred for cosmetic purposes due to its nongreasy and easily absorbable nature, but it is a more expensive oil too.

❋ *Flower-Infused Oil*

Ingredients

- ★ 1 cup oil of your choice
- ★ 7 grams of ground decarboxylated flower

Supplies

- ★ A slow cooker or double boiler
- ★ Candy thermometer
- ★ Spatula
- ★ Cheesecloth
- ★ Glass mason jar with lid

Pour the oil into the double boiler or slow cooker and add the ground flower, mixing extremely well. Ensure all the flower is fully saturated with the oil. Cook on low for 6–8 hours, stirring about every half an hour and checking the water level if you are using a double boiler. Be sure oil does not exceed 190°F. Let oil cool and then pour, straining through cheesecloth into the mason jar.

Flower-Infused Alcohol

There are two main reasons to infuse alcohol, the first being to make a tincture. Tinctures can be taken under the tongue (sublingually) for quick absorption into the bloodstream. Because of this, they have a high bioavailability and are fast acting. For sudden bouts of pain (like a sciatica flare up) tinctures can feel like a lifesaver. The effects of the alcohol help to calm nerves and relax your body and mind, allowing the CBD and other chemical constituents to get in and do their job. My tincture is my emergency kit. Sciatica flare? Tincture. Knee a table? Tincture. Throw out my back? Tincture. Sudden pain causes extra stress on the body. Tinctures help relieve the stress and the pain. To make a tincture, you want to use a base with a high alcohol content. I use Everclear. Remember, you will only be taking a dropper of this at a time. Not doing shots, a dropper. (Which means, yes, you do need a bottle with a dropper, preferably a brown, blue, or green bottle, as this helps protect the contents from light.)

While you can infuse alcohols on the stove, it is a fire hazard since they are extremely flammable. It is safer to use a slow cooker on low; or the safest bet yet is to use the jar process, though this one does take several weeks.

✺ *Slow Cooker Method for Everclear Tincture*

Ingredients

* ★ 1 cup oil of Everclear
* ★ 7 grams of ground decarboxylated flower

Supplies

* ★ A slow cooker or double boiler
* ★ Funnel
* ★ Cheesecloth
* ★ Brown, blue, or green (not clear) bottle with an eyedropper top

You want your tincture to be as strong and potent as can be by packing as much of the goodness that will come out of the flower into a small amount of alcohol. To do this, use 1 cup of Everclear with 7 grams of ground decarbed flower. Place it in the slow cooker and set to warm (this will keep your temperature around 160°F). Allow it to simmer for 30 minutes to an hour. After it cools, strain through cheesecloth and funnel into a bottle with an eyedropper top.

❄ *Jar Method for Everclear Tincture*

Ingredients

* ★ 7 grams of ground decarboxylated flower
* ★ 1 cup oil of Everclear

Supplies

* ★ Funnel
* ★ Cheesecloth
* ★ Glass mason jar with lid
* ★ Brown, blue, or green bottle with an eyedropper top

Place 7 grams of ground decarbed flower into the jar and cover with 1 cup of Everclear. Shake the jar gently and place in a warm location. You don't want it to get direct sunlight, but do not put it in a cold, dark place either. It needs to sit for 4 weeks, but you need to shake it every day, so the perfect location needs to be warm and visible so you don't forget about it. Mark the jar with the date you can stop shaking and strain through cheesecloth instead. Again, you will want to funnel it into a colored bottle with an eyedropper top.

You can infuse other alcohols too depending on your own personal tastes and what you want to use them for. Yes, it's perfectly acceptable to infuse vodka, rum, brandy, whisky—anything you want. A CBD-infused nightcap may be what helps you sleep at night. If you want to infuse any of the other alcohols as a tincture, you will follow the same process for using Everclear. However, if you want to infuse them for straight drinking or mixed cocktails, you do not need to use nearly as much flower. Instead of 7 grams to a cup, you can use 3.5 grams to 6 cups. You can still use the slow cooker method or use a large mason jar in the same way.

Flower-Infused Simple Syrup

Simple syrup is used in many cocktails. Therefore, you can add CBD to cocktails by infusing the syrup instead of infusing the alcohol, or you can infuse both. The sweetness of simple syrup does help counteract some of the flower taste too. This recipe is from Warren Bobrow's *Cannabis Cocktails, Mocktails & Tonics*.[52]

❀ *Flower-Infused Simple Syrup*

Ingredients

- ★ 2 cups water
- ★ 1 cup honey
- ★ 4 grams ground decarbed flower
- ★ 1 tbs liquid lecithin

....

52. Warren Bobrow, *Cannabis Cocktails, Mocktails & Tonics: The Art of Spirited Drinks & Buzz-Worthy Libations* (Beverly, MA: Fair Winds, 2016), 43.

Bring the water to a rolling boil in a saucepan, then reduce temperature until the water reaches 190°F. Stir in honey until it dissolves. Lower temperature again until the mixture cools to 160°F. Add flower, place a lid on the pan, and allow to simmer for a minimum of 30 minutes. Turn heat to low and add lecithin. Cook for 10 minutes longer while stirring constantly. Remove from the heat and strain through cheesecloth. Storing it in a dark colored glass bottle will allow it to stay fresh longer.

Save your plant material in an airtight container in the refrigerator for up to a week to use in some body care products we will visit later.

❀ *Flower-Infused Honey*
Infusing honey is another way to get CBD into your system, and it has skin care benefits, so it can be used in facial masks, soaps, and other body care products. The easiest, best, most effective way to infuse honey is with a slow cooker.

Ingredients

* ★ 7–14 grams of ground decarboxylated flower (depending on how strong you want to make it)

* ★ 2 cups honey (It is more difficult to work with less honey unless you have a mini slow cooker.)

Supplies

* ★ A slow cooker or double boiler

* ★ Spatula

- ★ Cheesecloth

- ★ Glass mason jar with lid

Tie up ground flower (not too fine) in cheesecloth and place in the bottom of the slow cooker. Pour the honey over the cheesecloth and set the slow cooker to warm. Every 20 minutes, stir the honey, scrape down the sides, and swirl the cheesecloth through the honey to help disperse everything throughout. Cook the honey for 5 hours. Scrape honey off the cheesecloth and set aside plant material to cool and save for other body care products recipes. Pour honey into a mason jar and allow to cool. You can do this with a double boiler, but you must make sure you keep the temperature below 160°F.

With these basic ingredients, there are many different recipes you can make. For starters, you can use these bases in any recipe you already use; however, do not forget that infusing anything with flower is going to alter the taste of it. When you first begin substituting, try before you commit. In other words, try in small doses first. Anything with a lot of flavor or spice is going to help cover the flower taste, so if you are someone who likes those types of foods, try your substitutions there first. Try it in things you bake too. The smaller the amount used, the less the overall taste of the final prepared dish will change, but you may notice a change in things you wouldn't expect. Some foods carry the flavor more intensely than others. It's going to be a bit of trial and error, but there's no rush. While many experiments will go great, you may have a few where you flat out say, "Ewww." I have learned I do not like scrambled eggs with infused butter, yet I am okay with a fried egg with infused butter. It's the weird little things we learn we like or don't like, and you will find them.

CHAPTER 5

The Body

When we think about how CBD helps the body, the first thing that usually comes to mind is the treatment of pain. This is one of the main uses for it. It can also be used in beauty and skin care products because of its properties. CBD helps clear up acne; it can be used on all skin types: dry, oily, or combination; it helps fill wrinkles; and it treats inflamed bags under the eyes. CBD has many uses; these are only a few.

In this chapter, we are going to talk about some of the great ways CBD can make your body feel great both inside and out. This chapter is going to focus on different recipes for both edible and skin care products. Let's start off by putting to use the plant material we saved after making some of our infusions.

❄️ *Ooey, Gooey Honey Facial Mask*

There's no point in wasting anything you don't have to, and the plant material left over from making the simple syrup and the infused honey are both going to have some honey and other goodness left in them you do not have to waste. Mix your used plant materials from these two infusions together and slowly add in a little more honey, stirring it into a thickened paste-like texture with the plant material fully coated. You don't want it to be runny. Tie your hair back or wrap it in a towel to keep it from getting in the way. Lie down and spread the honey-soaked plant material around your neck and face, avoiding the eye area. Maybe take a soak in a tub while you let it set. Soft music and aromatherapy oils in a diffuser can make this an even more relaxing task, and those are the best kinds of tasks to have! Give yourself a good 20–30 minutes at peace with this facial on. Use warm water to rinse the mask off (to help with any honey stickiness) followed by cool water.

A Word on Using Infused Oil versus CBD Concentrate

The oil-based recipes give you a choice between using CBD-infused jojoba oil (this is the oil you infused with plant material yourself) or using a CBD concentrate oil in your choice of strength. If you are using the concentrate, you will need to decide how much to add to your concoction. This is going to depend on how strong your concentrate is and how strong you want your final product to be. Obviously, the more you use, the stronger it will be. Generally, when I work with CBD concentrate oils, I will use a 1000 mg dosage and add 3–4 dropperfuls to my final mix. You may only need 1 dropperful. It really is going to be up to you. Some of the recipes come with recommendations as to what dosages to use, but always remember you can personalize them to work best for you. Experiment with different concentrations and amounts. This is something to keep track of, too, in your dosage journal.

✳ *Kerri's Jojoba Night Night Oil*

I refer to this as my Night Night Oil, because not only do I use it as part of my nightly facial care, but I also use it to help me wind down at night. The scents combine to be relaxing and peaceful while they fight dryness and wrinkles and tighten your facial skin. This does use jasmine oil, which can be on the pricey side. My suggestion? Go in on it with a friend or two. You will only be using a few drops at a time, so it can last quite a while, but if price is a concern, get some friends to buy it with you and then share or split into smaller dram bottles.

Ingredients

- ⋆ 4 oz. of flower-infused jojoba oil, or 4 oz. of jojoba oil and a CBD concentrate oil in your choice of strength
- ⋆ 4 oz. bottle (check your local dollar store)
- ⋆ 8 drops jasmine essential oil
- ⋆ 4 drops lavender essential oil
- ⋆ 2 drops frankincense essential oil

Add the jojoba oil to the 4 oz. bottle about ¾ of the way full, leaving enough room for the other ingredients—you can top off with more jojoba oil if you need to. If it is not already infused, add CBD concentrated oil in the strength of your choice. Add the jasmine, lavender, and frankincense oils. If you really want to stretch out your jasmine oil, switch the number of drops with the lavender oil. This will give you a different scent but will still work well with your skin and your sleep. Top off with more jojoba if needed and be sure to shake well before each use. At night, right before bed, use only a few drops, spreading them gently over your face and neck. Breathe in the scent and allow your body and mind to relax and drift off to sleep.

Oooooh, That Feels Good Muscle Pain Relief Massage Oil

One of the things you learn when dealing with chronic pain is there are many different types of pain. These different types of pain respond to different treatments. Muscle pain is not the same as inflammation pain, and yes, you may have one without the other, or sometimes you may have both, but they will be in different parts of the body. For example, when I first started doing my best to hit my daily step goal, not only did my knees end up with a lot of inflammation, but my calves were also suffering too. These are different types of pain I know I can treat differently for maximum results.

Ingredients

* ⋆ 4 oz. of flower-infused jojoba oil, or 4 oz. of jojoba oil and a CBD concentrate oil in your choice of strength

* ⋆ 4 oz. bottle

* ⋆ 8 drops marjoram essential oil

* ⋆ 6 drops peppermint essential oil

* ⋆ 4 drops basil essential oil

* ⋆ 4 drops wintergreen essential oil

* ⋆ 3 drops bergamot essential oil

Add the jojoba oil to the 4 oz. bottle, leaving enough room for the other ingredients—you can top off with more jojoba oil if you need to. If it is not already infused, add CBD concentrated oil in the strength of your choice. Add the essential oils. Top off with more jojoba if needed and be sure to shake well before each use. This can also be used with a roller-ball top on your bottle. Use on tight, sore, overworked, strained muscles by massaging in deeply.

❀ *My Aching Joints Inflammation Relief Oil*

I have osteoarthritis in my knees; they swell terribly, and they pop and crack with every step. I have had large needles inserted into them to drain off fluid before, and let me tell you, it is plain awful. It's excruciating. When I decided to start trying a more natural approach to my health care, the next time my knees needed draining, I took a pass to see if anything else would work. I did research on some different therapies. While I do still use acupuncture to help, using this oil when I start feeling the swelling come on keeps the worst of it at bay and often wipes it out in a couple of days altogether.

Ingredients

* ★ 4 oz. of flower-infused jojoba oil, or 4 oz. of jojoba oil and a CBD concentrate oil in your choice of strength

* ★ 4 oz. bottle

* ★ 3 drops oregano essential oil

* ★ 3 drops nutmeg essential oil

* ★ 3 drops lemongrass essential oil

* ★ 3 drops dill essential oil

* ★ 3 drops peppermint essential oil

* ★ 8 drops tangerine essential oil

Add the jojoba oil to the 4 oz. bottle about ½ of the way full, leaving enough room for the other ingredients. If it is not already infused, add CBD concentrated oil in the strength of your choice. Add the essential oils. Top off with more jojoba to fill the bottle. Be sure to shake well before each use and massage sparingly into the inflamed area.

Bath Salt Recipes

Adding bath salts to your bath are a great way to get healing benefits from the salt, hot water, CBD, and essential oils used. These recipes have been provided by Krystle Hope, owner of Crescent Sapphire.

When using herbs in a bath salt blend, it is important to grind the herbs using an herb grinder or food processer to avoid clogging any bathtub drains. Alternatively, a mesh tub strainer or cheesecloth could be used to trap larger herbs to be tossed out instead of clogging the drain.

✸ *Bath Salts for Soothing Sore Muscles*

Ingredients

* ★ 3 cups Epsom salts (magnesium sulfate)
* ★ ½ cup pink Himalayan salt
* ★ ½ cup Dead Sea salt
* ★ ¼ cup baking soda
* ★ 10 drops clove essential oil, or 1 tsp clove powder (do not use whole cloves)
* ★ 10 drops eucalyptus essential oil
* ★ 10 drops rosemary essential oil, or ¼ cup dried rosemary
* ★ Up to 2 ml of CBD concentrated oil of your choice

Blend the salts and baking soda together first. Add in essential and CBD oils, blending well and using a fork to break up any lumps. Add in dried rosemary, if using, and blend again. Store in an airtight container.

✳ *Bath Salts for Easing Inflammation*

Ingredients

- ★ 3 cups Epsom salts (magnesium sulfate)
- ★ ½ cup pink Himalayan salt
- ★ ½ cup Dead Sea salt
- ★ ¼ cup baking soda
- ★ 15 drops tangerine essential oil
- ★ 10 drops thyme essential oil
- ★ 10 drops tulsi basil essential oil (also called holy basil or tulsi), or ¼ cup of the dried herb
- ★ Up to 2 ml of CBD concentrated oil of your choice

Blend the salts and baking soda together first. Add in essential and CBD oils, blending well and using a fork to break up any lumps. Add in dried basil, if using, and blend again. Store in an airtight container.

✳ *Moisturizing Beard Oil*

This recipe was provided to us by Cheryl's associate and friend Jolanta Chalupczak, formerly from Peaceful Waters CBD Shop. CBD has great moisturizing capabilities that, when combined with jojoba, make for a supple and soft beard.

Ingredients

* ★ 20 ml jojoba oil

* ★ 100 mg CBD[53]

* ★ 3 drops lavender essential oil

* ★ 2 drops peppermint essential oil

Mix all ingredients in a 1 oz. (30 ml) dropper bottle or larger. You will only need a drop or two at a time depending on beard length.

Smoking Blends

If you smoke CBD flower, blends are a fun way to add terpenes, flavor, and more benefits to your practice. Ensure the ingredients you use to create your blends are food grade. Do not smoke flowers from a florist. The last place you want all the fertilizers and chemicals that go into florist's flowers is in your lungs.

You can make simple blends by adding single herbs or other items to your CBD flower or more complex blends by combining two or more. Take the flavor of the individual items you are using into account before combining herbs together for your own mixes but do make up some of your own mixes. Try different things and see what you like. It can

....

53. We prefer using 1.5 ml of the 2000 mg/30 ml CBD isolate tincture.

become quite the hobby learning about the benefits of the different herbs and mixing them into healing, smokable combinations. For example, peppermint and thyme aren't going to taste particularly good together, but lavender and jasmine do. Also, before smoking anything, be sure it is something that you can smoke without it making you sick or worse. While many plants can be smoked, some will kill you if you try. Know which is which.

When you are using a blend, you want it to accent, not overpower, your flower. To ensure a good distribution, mix your blends and do not add your CBD flower until you are ready to smoke it. A mortar and pestle help to ensure well-mixed blends. (I know many people love marble sets, but I have found wood ones to work just as well if not better.)

After mixing your blends together, store them in airtight containers until ready for use. Then, blend them with your CBD flower. You may want to go as high as a fifty-fifty mix, but this is entirely up to you, and it will depend on the blend you are using. Remember, the less CBD flower you use, the less CBD you will consume.

❀ Pain Relief Smoking Blend
Cinnamon, cloves, and hops are all high in beta-caryophyllene. This terpene is an anti-inflammatory and works well to relieve neuropathy and arthritic pain.

You will want to use this particular blend in a small ration compared to your CBD. Hops can be pricey, so this may also be a factor in how far you want this blend to stretch.

Cinnamon and clove are also very potent, and you will be using them in a ground form. I recommend trying this blend first at about 20 percent and 80 percent CBD flower. If you like it, you can go for a stronger mix.

Ingredients

- ⋆ 1 cup dried ground hops (you may have to grind them yourself)
- ⋆ 2 tbs ground cinnamon
- ⋆ 1 tbs ground clove

Thoroughly blend the mixture together. It won't be overly pretty, as the cinnamon and clove will coat the hops with a thick dusting. Before combining with your CBD flower, be sure to give its jar a good shake again, and let it settle a moment before opening so you don't get a face full of cinnamon and clove cloud.

I Just Want to Sleep Insomnia Relief Smoking Blend

Rich in the sleep aid linalool, this blend will also help to calm anxiety and promote the feeling of being at peace.

It has several ingredients, so we will only be using a small amount of each. If we didn't, you would need a gallon-size container to store it!

Ingredients

- ⋆ ¼ cup lavender
- ⋆ ¼ cup chamomile

* ¼ cup hops

* ¼ cup jasmine flowers

* ¼ cup lemon balm

* ¼ cup mugwort

* ¼ cup skullcap

After mixing the ingredients, grind them together with a mortar and pestle or in an electric grinder if you would like a finer grind. Grinding the herbs together and blending them again ensures the most efficient distribution of each herb—important to do when you are blending several types of herbs together. You want to ensure every dose has a little bit of everything. A fine grind helps. Smooth taste with a nice aroma, this blend will help you sleep through the night and relax in peaceful dreams.

✸ I'm All Stuffed Up Congestion Relief Smoking Blend

Head cold, chest cold, upper respiratory infection, sinus infections. All of these can be treated with this blend. (And a visit to your doctor when needed. Always remember, CBD is in addition to medical care, not instead of it. Infections can be serious business and should be treated as such.)

Ingredients

* ¼ cup coltsfoot

* ¼ cup echinacea

* ¼ cup eucalyptus

* ¼ cup mullein

* ¼ cup peppermint

After mixing the ingredients, grind them together with a mortar and pestle or in an electric grinder if you would like a finer grind. Packed with healing herbs, this blend helps clear your head and lungs.

Tantalizing Temptations

Finding ways to incorporate CBD into your daily routine with tasty recipes is key to success. If you aren't enjoying what you are eating, it makes it difficult to build new, healthier eating habits. These recipes help you add CBD in fun, healthy, and delicious ways.

✸ Eye-Opener Citrus Smoothie Blast

Starting your day off with a CBD-infused Citrus Smoothie Blast helps you focus; it's energizing and eye opening, helping you to feel refreshed and ready to go. This smoothie combines the terpene limonene from several different sources. It is a bit of a process to make because you will be doing your own juicing too, but because the juice can be refrigerated for several days, you do not have to juice daily. You can juice twice a week to add this incredibly healthy kick to your diet.

You will need a zester. The peels of citrus fruits are high in limonene, but you do not want to juice the entire peel, as it will end up tasting very bitter. Instead, we are going to zest off parts of the peel and store those separately to add to the smoothies. Resealable plastic bags work great for storing the zest. Store each zest in a different bag; what you don't use in your smoothies can be used in other ways, including added to bath water, into a muslin bag to add to your shower, or even to a vinegar water solution to use as a cleanser.

You need a blender capable of crushing ice.

Ingredients

* **Juice base:**

    * 1 organic lemon

    * 1 organic lime

    * 8 organic oranges

* **Per each smoothie:**

    * 1 cup juice base

    * 1 tbs CBD-infused coconut oil or your preferred dosage of concentrate oil

    * 1 banana

    * 1 cup Greek yogurt

    * 1 cup ice

    * Optional: sweetener of your choice

Utensils

* Zester

* Juicer

* Blender

After zesting as much of the lemon, lime, and orange as you want (there will be other ways to use dried zest in later recipes), peel each fruit and juice, combining the lemon, lime, and orange juices together. This part can be stored in the refrigerator for four days. When you are ready to prepare a smoothie, use 1 cup of the juice, the coconut or CBD oil, 1 banana cut in chunks, and 1 cup Greek yogurt in a blender with any sweetener of your choosing. Blend, giving the coconut oil the opportunity to blend in before adding ice, which will make the coconut chunk up if not well blended in first. Once it is ready, add in ice and blend again.

❄ Inflammation-Busting Juice

I hate inflammation. I truly do. There aren't many things I hate, but inflammation is one of them. A problem that used to only exist in my larger joints eventually made its way to my smaller ones. Since I don't take pharmaceuticals and hardly any over-the-counter meds even, I have had to find other ways to control my inflammation, particularly on days when I am having a flare. Those of us who deal with autoimmune issues understand there are all kinds of triggers that can throw our immune systems into attack mode, so though we try to control as much as we can, flares happen and have to be tapered down.

This is the recipe I use when I am in a flare and need help getting things back under control. Celery and cucumber are both excellent at fighting inflammation, and they help to flush our systems. Combined with the inflammation-fighting terpene pinene found in the basil, this juice helps to pack a potent punch.

Because I don't like juicing every day, I make enough for three days, which is generally enough time to get my immune system to sit back down and behave and rid myself of the extra swelling affecting my joints.

Ingredients

*   ★ 1 bunch of organic celery

*   ★ A handful of fresh basil leaves

*   ★ 4 organic cucumbers (I leave the peels on, but if you really don't like to juice your peels, by all means, peel them.)

*   ★ 1 tbs CBD-infused coconut oil or your preferred dosage of concentrate oil

I begin by juicing the celery, then the basil leaves, and finally the cucumber last; since it is the "juiciest," it helps clean up the machine a little bit. Add all the juices to one large pitcher. Always be sure to stir before serving. Add the CBD to your individual serving, not to the pitcher of juice. I like to blend it well in the large pitcher and then pour into shaker bottles with mixing balls. This makes it easy for me to grab, shake, and go.

❁ Amp'd Easy Box Brownies
From Cheryl Cryer

These easy-to-make brownies use a regular box of brownie mix as a base but add in extra cocoa and espresso to give it an extra-chocolatey rich taste.

Serving size: 1 brownie square
CBD per serving: 10 mg
Servings per batch: 16
CBD per batch: 160 mg

Ingredients

* ★ 2 eggs

* ★ 1 stick (½ cup) unsalted butter, melted

* ★ ⅓ cup buttermilk or milk

* ★ 160 mg CBD oil[54]

* ★ 18.3 oz. brownie mix

* ★ ¼ cup cocoa powder

* ★ 1 tsp espresso powder (optional, but makes chocolate flavor richer and will not taste like coffee)

Preheat oven to 325°F. Line an 8 x 8-inch square pan with parchment paper and spray with nonstick cooking spray. Set aside.

Combine the eggs, melted butter, milk, and CBD oil in a mixing bowl and beat with an electric mixer for a minute.

Add brownie mix, cocoa powder, and espresso powder and blend again for another minute.

....

54. Note: We prefer using the 5000 mg/30 ml full-spectrum CBD oil (see appendix) for infusing due to the concentration, which would be 1 ml per batch. For lower-concentrated CBD oils, do not use more than 3 ml of oil per batch, or adjust the liquids accordingly. Alternately, you can use CBD isolate powder.

Pour the brownie batter into the prepared pan, spreading evenly with a spatula.

Bake for 50 minutes or until a toothpick inserted in the center comes out clean. Allow the brownies to cool. Remove the brownies from the pan using the parchment paper. Slice and serve. Store in an airtight container. Do not refrigerate.

❄ *Chocolate Lollipops*

From Cheryl Cryer

Serving size: 1 lollipop
CBD per serving: 5 mg
Servings per batch: 16
CBD per batch: 80 mg

Ingredients

* ★ 8 oz. dark chocolate for melting (or mix it up: 4 oz. white and 4 oz. dark or milk)

* ★ 80 mg CBD oil[55]

* ★ Sprinkles or toppings such as crushed nuts (optional)

* ★ Lollipop molds

* ★ Lollipop sticks

* ★ Cellophane and ties for packaging

....

55. Note: We prefer using the 5000 mg/30 ml full-spectrum CBD oil (see appendix) for infusing due to the concentration, which would be 0.5 ml per batch. For lower-concentrated CBD oils, do not use more than 1 ml of oil per batch or the chocolate won't set up. Alternately, you can use CBD isolate powder premixed with 1 ml of canola or fractionated coconut oil.

Melt dark chocolate slowly either using a double boiler or in the microwave in 30-second bursts. Stir frequently.

Add CBD oil into the melted dark chocolate and mix well. Pour the melted chocolate into your lollipop molds and add lollipop stick. Add optional sprinkles or toppings.

Place in the refrigerator for a few hours until chocolate is solid.

Carefully remove from lollipop molds by easing the mold away from the chocolate and not pulling on the stick.

Wrap and tie for storing or giving to family and friends to introduce them to the wonderful world of CBD.

Pumpkin Spice Granola Bars

From Cheryl Cryer

Serving size: 1 bar
CBD per serving: 10 mg
Servings per batch: 10
CBD per batch: 100 mg

Ingredients

* ★ 2 cups old-fashioned rolled oats
* ★ 1 cup brown rice crisp cereal
* ★ ¼ cup dried cranberries
* ★ 2–3 tbs pepitas
* ★ ½ cup honey
* ★ ½ cup coconut oil (measured when liquid)

* 100 mg CBD oil[56]

* 1 tsp pumpkin pie spice

* ½ tsp vanilla

* ¼ tsp sea salt

Line an 8 x 8-inch square baking pan with parchment.

Combine oats, cereal, ⅛ cup of dried cranberries, and 1 tbs of pepitas in a large mixing bowl. Set aside.

Over medium heat, combine honey and coconut oil in a pot. Stirring continuously, let it bubble for 30 seconds. Remove from heat and stir in CBD oil, pumpkin pie spice, vanilla, and sea salt.

Pour honey mixture into dry ingredients and mix until well coated. Pour into baking pan and lightly press to ensure it is even.

Top with remaining dried cranberries and pepitas and press down firmly (with a piece of parchment paper) as much as possible. (Skipping this step may result in crumbly bars.)

Place pan in the refrigerator for a couple hours. Once bars are hard to the touch, remove from pan and place on a cutting board. Slice into 10 bars. Serve immediately or store in an airtight container for up to one week.

....

56. Note: We prefer using the 5000 mg/30 ml full-spectrum CBD oil (see appendix) for infusing due to the concentration, which would be 0.6 ml per batch. For lower-concentrated CBD oils, do not use more than 2 ml of oil per batch and adjust the coconut oil accordingly. Alternatively, you can use CBD isolate powder.

✸ *Classic Caramel Corn*

From Cheryl Cryer

Serving size: 1 cup
CBD per serving: 10 mg
Servings per batch: 10 cups
CBD per batch: 100 mg

Ingredients

- ★ 10 cups of popped popcorn
- ★ Salt to taste
- ★ 1 cup sweet cream salted butter
- ★ 2 cups light brown sugar
- ★ 2 tsp vanilla
- ★ ½ tsp baking soda
- ★ 100 mg CBD oil[57]

Pop popcorn, removing any un-popped kernels. Salt popcorn as desired and set aside.

Melt the butter in a medium saucepan over medium heat. Pour in the brown sugar and stir thoroughly. Bring the butter and sugar mixture up to a boil on medium heat, stirring continuously, and cook for an additional 4 minutes. Add in vanilla;

....

57. Note: We prefer using the 5000 mg/30 ml full-spectrum CBD oil (see appendix) for infusing due to the concentration, which would be 0.6 ml per batch. For lower-concentrated CBD oils, do not use more than 3 ml of oil per batch or adjust the liquids accordingly. Alternately, you can use CBD isolate powder.

stir for one more minute. Add in the baking soda and stir, continuing to boil for one last minute and then remove from heat. Add CBD and mix thoroughly.

Carefully fold in caramel mixture to popped popcorn, ensuring all kernels are covered. Spread the popcorn out onto a cookie sheet lined with parchment paper and allow to cool before serving.

❀ No Bake Energy Bites
From Cheryl Cryer
Serving size: 1 energy bite
CBD per serving: 15 mg
Servings per batch: 14
CBD per batch: 210 mg

Ingredients

* ½ cup creamy peanut butter

* ⅓ cup honey

* 1 tsp vanilla extract

* ⅔ cup toasted shredded coconut (sweetened or unsweetened)

* 1 cup old-fashioned oats

* ½ cup ground flaxseed

* ½ cup semisweet chocolate chips (or vegan chocolate chips)

* 1 tbs chia seeds (optional)

* 210 mg CBD oil[58]

In a large bowl, stir everything together, starting with wet ingredients first and then combining in the dry. Mix well, ensuring the dry ingredients are fully covered.

Cover bowl and chill in the refrigerator for 1–2 hours. Once mixture is thoroughly chilled, roll into 1-inch balls.

Enjoy immediately or refrigerate in a sealed container for up to one week (or freeze for up to 3 months).

Sugarless, Flourless Oat Cookies

From Cheryl Cryer
Serving size: 1 cookie
CBD per serving: 10 mg
Servings per batch: 12 cookies
CBD per batch: 120 mg

Ingredients

* 3 bananas

* 80 mg CBD oil[59]

....

58. Note: We prefer using the 5000 mg/30 ml full-spectrum CBD oil (see appendix) for infusing due to the concentration, which would be 1.26 ml per batch. For lower-concentrated CBD oils, do not use more than 2 ml of oil per batch or the chocolate won't set up. Alternately, you can use CBD isolate powder mixed with up to 2 ml of fractionated coconut oil.

59. Note: We prefer using the 5000 mg/30 ml full-spectrum CBD oil (see appendix) for infusing due to the concentration, which would be 0.75 ml per batch. For lower-concentrated CBD oils, do not use more than 1 ml of oil per batch or the mixture may not set up. Alternately, you can use CBD isolate powder premixed with 1 ml of canola or fractionated coconut oil.

* 1¾ cups rolled oats

* ½ cup date sugar

* 2 pinches cinnamon

* 1 tsp vanilla

* ½ cup dark chocolate

Preheat oven to 325°F.

In a large bowl, mash the bananas with a fork or masher until no chunks remain. Add the CBD oil in and blend thoroughly. Fold in rolled oats and date sugar and again blend thoroughly. Stir in cinnamon and vanilla.

Spoon the batter into 12 mounds on a parchment-lined baking sheet. Bake for 15–20 minutes until the outsides become golden and solid. Remove from the oven to cool.

While the cookies are cooling, in a small bowl, heat dark chocolate chips in the microwave for 20 seconds at a time, stirring frequently until melted and smooth. Drizzle dark chocolate over the cookies while they are still cooling.

Once cool, store in an airtight container in the refrigerator for up to one week.

CHAPTER 6

The Mind

We know CBD is great for physical ailments and to help the body function at its best level, but what about the mind? How does CBD affect it? Many people are afraid that CBD will be like its counterpart THC and give you a "high" feeling. This is a falsehood and simply not true. CBD will never get you high.

There are things it can do for your mind. It can help calm your nerves. It can help lift depression. It can pack up anxiety and ship it away. It can not only help you get to sleep at night, but can also help you stay asleep. Some people are now using it to treat seizures and Parkinson's disease (under the guide of a doctor of course). In what ways can CBD help you?

Tea

When buying ingredients to use in making teas, always ensure you are getting food grade. You will be able to find some things at your local grocery store or gourmet grocery store. Other items you may have to search for online. You do not want to be using products that are covered in pesticides or other chemicals. I know many people who want to save flowers from the florists to use for other things later; this is fine, but do not consume florist flowers in any manner. They are covered in chemicals, often including glues and varnishes, not to mention the massive amount of fertilizers and pesticides. Use them in potpourri if you like, but don't eat or smoke them and don't use them in products to use on your skin.

Mix up the dry ingredients for each tea recipe in a large bowl, being sure to blend extremely well before storing in an airtight resealable container. Corked glass jars are great for holding tea blends. If you are using dried CBD flower, mix it in with the dry ingredients. If you are adding CBD concentrate to your tea, you can do that after you have it brewed and are ready to drink.

When preparing teas to drink, use hot but not boiling water. For an 8 oz. cup, add 2–3 teaspoons of your chosen tea blend to a mesh ball strainer or tea bag. Adjust measurement and sweetness to taste.

❂ *It's All Groovy Anxiety Relief Tea*

* ⋆ 1 cup dried lavender buds

* ⋆ 1 cup dried lemon balm

* ⋆ 1 cup dried CBD flower (if using)

❂ *Bull's-Eye Blast Focus Tea*

* ⋆ 1 cup dried crushed sage leaves

* ⋆ 1 cup dried CBD flower (if using)

* ⋆ ½ cup dried ginger root (chopped, not finely ground)

* ⋆ ½ cup dried crushed lemon peel

If you have any leftover lemon zest, you can dry it and add it to this tea too for an extra lemony taste and an extra boost of limonene. Honey makes the perfect sweetener for this tea if you can use it, as the flavor blends so well with the dried ingredients.

❂ *La-La Land Nighttime Sleep Tea*

* ⋆ 2 cups dried chamomile buds

* ⋆ 1 cup dried lavender buds

* ⋆ 1 cup dried CBD flower (if using)

* ⋆ ½ cup chopped dried mango

❀ Mood Booster Uplifting Tea

This is another tea where you can use your extra zest and citrus rinds that you have dried and saved, and it will have some caffeine to give you an extra kick.

- ★ 1 cup chamomile buds
- ★ 1 cup green tea leaves
- ★ 1 cup dried CBD flower (if using)
- ★ ¼ cup dried crushed lemon peels
- ★ ⅛ cup dried crushed lime peels
- ★ ¼ cup dried crushed orange peels

Add up to a tablespoon of each: dried lemon zest, dried lime zest, dried orange zest. Or up to 3 tablespoons in any combination (2 orange and 1 lemon, for example). Adjust to your own personal taste and consider what you have on hand.

❀ Zen Meditation Tea

- ★ 1 cup dried chamomile flowers
- ★ ½ cup dried mugwort
- ★ ½ cup dried lemon balm
- ★ 1 cup dried CBD flower (if using)

❀ Oooooh, Honey Aphrodisiac Tea

- ★ ½ cup dried damiana
- ★ ½ cup dried hibiscus

- ★ ½ cup dried jasmine flowers

- ★ ½ cup dried blue lotus flowers

- ★ 1 cup dried CBD flower (if using)

Oils

Oils are one of my favorite ingredients to work with because it really is very easy to mix up your own. They are also easy to use as either a massage oil or to apply to pulse points for aromatherapy benefits. These next recipes can be made up and stored as a part of your "medicine cabinet" so that they are always ready and on hand when you need them. Remember, carrier oils will eventually spoil and go rancid. Be sure to check the expiration date on your carrier oil, and be sure to mark your newly concocted potions with the expiration date and the name of the oil so as to not confuse what they are.

✼ *Let It Go Tension Relief Oil*

Bad day at work? Kids driving you crazy? Many people report feeling calmer after using a CBD-infused oil on their skin. This tension relief oil is great to help you unwind and relax when you are particularly stressed out.

Ingredients

- ★ 4 oz. of flower-infused jojoba oil, or 4 oz. of jojoba oil and a CBD supplement oil in your choice of strength

- ★ 4 oz. bottle

- ★ 10 drops lavender oil

- ★ 2 drops orange oil

- ★ 2 drops lemon oil

- ★ 2 drops chamomile oil

- ★ 2 drops ylang-ylang oil

Add the jojoba oil to the 4 oz. bottle about halfway, leaving enough room for the other ingredients—you can top off with more jojoba oil if you need to. If it is not already infused, add CBD concentrated oil in the strength of your choice. Add the essential oils.

When needed, shake well and apply to pulse points, neck, and your temples. Take several deep breaths as you calm and unwind. If you are holding tension in your body—tightened shoulders, clenched jaw—rub this oil into these areas to help them relax.

☼ Deep State Meditation Oil

This meditation oil should be used when you are getting ready to go into a meditative state. While of course you can have someone else put it on you, it is also an incredibly positive experience to apply it yourself before meditation. Self-massage is a perfect way to learn more about your own body and how it feels and responds to touch. It can also be a bit of its own meditation as you focus on applying the oil and taking in its scent.

You can mix the essential oils listed together without the carrier oil to add to a diffuser during meditation if you like.

This is a blend I recently created, and I am in love with it for my meditation practices.

Ingredients

* 4 oz. of flower-infused jojoba oil, or 4 oz. of jojoba oil and a CBD supplement oil in your choice of strength
* 4 oz. bottle
* 5 drops amber oil
* 5 drops frankincense oil
* 5 drops lavender oil
* 2 drops patchouli oil

Add the jojoba oil to the 4 oz. bottle about ⅔ of the way, leaving enough room for the other ingredients—you can top off with more jojoba oil if you need to. If it is not already infused, add CBD concentrated oil in the strength of your choice. Then add the essential oils. Be sure to shake well before use. Apply to neck, temples, and any pulse points you like. You can also use this to massage your arms to help take in the scent before you perform your meditation.

✺ Slow Wave Deep Sleep Oil

The insomniac that I am, I use several different methods to help me sleep at night. This oil is for when I need a good, deep, restful sleep. If I try to sleep "cold," as in with no help, I average about three hours of sleep. My general sleep routine, and what my body is used to, runs me an average of five hours a night. Eventually, I do get worn out, and when I do and need a deep sleep to help me recharge, this massage oil gets added into the routine.

Why don't I use it every day if it helps me sleep more than five hours at a time? I am used to five hours of sleep and that gives me a nineteen-hour day, so I have plenty of time to get things done. On the rare occasion when I do sleep in and get eight hours or more of rest, I also lose hours in the day.

This oil will help you relax and get the sleep your body and mind need. You can also mix the essential oils listed together without the carrier oil to add to a diffuser to help you sleep.

Ingredients

* 4 oz. of flower-infused jojoba oil, or 4 oz. of jojoba oil and a CBD supplement oil in your choice of strength

* 4 oz. bottle

* 6 drops bergamot

* 5 drops chamomile

* 5 drops lavender

* 3 drops dill

Add the jojoba oil to the 4 oz. bottle, leaving enough room for the other ingredients—you can top off with more jojoba oil if you need to. If it is not already infused, add CBD concentrated oil in the strength of your choice. Add in the essential oils. Shake well before each use and massage all over the body before bed.

Bath Soaks

Bath soaks are normally a relaxing activity all on their own, but when you add CBD to the mix, you add in extra benefits. CBD oil is moisturizing and nurturing. It will make your skin feel smooth and supple. CBD will also help relax muscles and ease pain. Combine these effects with those achieved through aromatherapy, and it is easy to see why CBD in the tub has become so popular.

❋ *Cheerful Blend CBD Bath Soak*
From Cheryl Cryer

Ingredients

* ★ 5 drops grapefruit essential oil

* ★ 30 mg CBD oil[60]

* ★ ½ cup pink Himalayan salt (You can replace with any bath salt like Epsom salts or pure magnesium flakes.)

Combine essential oil and CBD oil in a glass bowl. Add salt and mix well. Pour into a hot bath and soak for 20–30 minutes for best results.

....

60. Note: We prefer using the 1000 mg/30 ml full-spectrum CBD oil for this single recipe, which would be 1 ml (1 dropperful) in this concentration. Alternately, you can use CBD isolate powder premixed with 1ml fractionated coconut oil.

❊ Cheerful Blend Melt and Pour Soap

From Cheryl Cryer

Soap size: 4 oz.

CBD per soap: 50 mg

Soap per batch: 6

CBD per batch: 300 mg

Ingredients

* ⋆ 5 ml grapefruit essential oil

* ⋆ 300 mg CBD oil[61]

* ⋆ Mica colorant (optional)

* ⋆ 3 cups melt and pour soap base

* ⋆ 6-cavity soap mold (4 oz. each cavity)

* ⋆ Alcohol in a spray bottle

In a 4-cup pourable glass mixing cup, mix together the essential oil, CBD, and mica colorant and set aside.

Melt the soap base using a double boiler or in the microwave (half power, stirring every 60 seconds). Stir frequently.

Partially pour the soap base into your oil mixture and stir. If using mica, make sure it is thoroughly mixed. Add remaining soap base and mix again.

....

61. Note: We prefer using the 5000 mg/30 ml full-spectrum CBD oil (see appendix) for infusing due to the high concentration, which would be 1.8 ml per batch. Alternately, you can use CBD isolate powder premixed with no more than 2 ml of fractionated coconut oil.

Spray your soap molds with alcohol. Pour the hot melted soap into molds and spray the tops again with alcohol. Allow to cool completely before removing.

✿ *Stress Relief Bath Salts*
From Krystle Hope of Crescent Sapphire

Ingredients

* ★ 3 cups Epsom salts (magnesium sulfate)
* ★ ½ cup pink Himalayan salt
* ★ ½ cup Dead Sea salt
* ★ Up to 2 ml CBD concentrate oil of your choice
* ★ ¼ cup lavender flowers
* ★ ¼ cup chamomile flowers or tea
* ★ Optional: Up to 20 drops of your favorite relaxing essential oils such as lavender, chamomile, geranium, ylang-ylang, or neroli

Blend the salts together first. If adding essential oils, mix them with the CBD oil first and then blend well, using a fork to break up any lumps. Add in dried flowers and blend again. Store in an airtight container.

✿ *Aromatherapy Bath Bombs*

This bath bomb recipe is from Cheryl's friend and associate Jolanta Chalupczak, formerly of Peaceful Waters CBD Shop. This is a base recipe, meaning you can choose which essential oils you would like to use in it.

Bath bomb size: 2.5 inches
CBD per bath bomb: 65 mg
Bath bombs per batch: 9
CBD per batch: 585 mg

Dry ingredients

- ⋆ 2 cups baking soda

- ⋆ 1 cup Epsom salts

- ⋆ 1 cup corn starch

- ⋆ 1 cup citric acid

Wet ingredients

- ⋆ 60 ml (2 oz.) coconut oil

- ⋆ 585 mg CBD oil[62]

- ⋆ 7 ml essential oils of your choice (For a mood lifting blend, we recommend mixing equal amounts orange, peppermint, and frankincense.)

Utensils

- ⋆ Plastic gloves

- ⋆ Molds for bath bombs

Begin by mixing the dry ingredients together thoroughly in a large bowl. Set aside. Combine the wet ingredients together first in a separate bowl and then add to the dry ingredients.

....

62. We prefer using 8.7 ml of the 2000 mg/30 ml CBD isolate tincture.

Wear gloves to thoroughly mix together and knead until there are no lumps and the mixture feels like wet sand. Pack the ingredients into molds and allow to dry overnight in an area with low humidity. Once they have hardened, remove from mold and wrap in plastic wrap to keep dry.

Smoking Blends

Remember, when using a blend, the goal is to compliment not overpower your flower. To ensure a good distribution, mix your blends without the CBD flower until you are ready to smoke it. When ready to add CBD flower, again you may want to go as high as a fifty-fifty mix, but it is entirely up to you, and it will depend on the blend you are using. Remember, the less CBD flower you use, the less CBD you will consume.

❋ Calming

This calming blend will help you relax, whether after a long day at work or if your anxiety is high. This will soothe the nerves and relax the mind.

Ingredients

- ★ ¼ cup blue vervain
- ★ ¼ cup hops
- ★ ¼ cup lotus flower
- ★ ¼ cup passionflower

Mix and grind the ingredients together to the fineness you desire and store in an airtight glass jar. All of these plants have known calming properties and are great for mellowing you out when you are overstressed.

❀ *Energizing*

When you want an energetic pick-me-up, use a mix of peppermint and holy basil.

Ingredients

* ★ 1 cup peppermint

* ★ ½ cup holy basil

Mix and grind the ingredients to the desired fineness. Adjust the mixture to taste if you need. Both herbs are great for an energy boost. Peppermint contains limonene, so it is energizing and uplifting along with helping you focus. (Which is why it is in the next smoking blend too.)

❀ *Focus*

I am sure if I were a child today, I would be diagnosed with ADHD. I have learned to adjust to my distractable nature, though, having dealt with it for so many years now. This blend helps calm the mind from other distractions and helps you to concentrate and focus.

Ingredients

* ★ 1 cup peppermint

* ★ ¼ cup hyssop

* ¼ cup skullcap

* ¼ cup morning glory

Mix ingredients together and grind to the desired fineness. As always, store the blend in an airtight glass container.

Chill Out with Chocolate

If you are working with a CBD oil, incorporating it into desserts, especially chocolate, is a brilliant way to help counteract the earthy flavor of the concentrate. Chocolate candies also make for an easy and enjoyable way to dose. While this will also work for people taking CBD for pain, it can be an extra special way to relax while reducing anxiety and stress. Whether you want to curl up in some jammies and chill or soak in a warm CBD-infused aromatherapy bath, chocolate is often a welcome guest to help soothe the soul. When the chocolate contains CBD to calm your nerves and mind, it's even better.

These wonderful chocolate recipes were provided by Cheryl's friend and associate Lori Smerz from The Party Kitchen.

❀ *Dark Chocolate CBD Bark*
(With Variations: Peppermint/Strawberry)

From Lori Smerz

Serving size: 1 oz.

CBD per serving: 7.5 mg

Servings per batch: 32

CBD per batch: 240 mg

Ingredients

- ★ 16 oz. dark chocolate for melting
- ★ 240 mg CBD oil[63]
- ★ ½ tsp pure peppermint or strawberry extract
- ★ ½ cup (halved) crushed peppermint candies or dehydrated strawberries
- ★ 16 oz. white chocolate for melting
- ★ Double boiler or microwave
- ★ Parchment paper
- ★ Cookie sheet or sheet pan

Melt the dark chocolate slowly either using a double boiler or in the microwave in 30-second bursts. Stir frequently. Add CBD oil and extract into the melted dark chocolate and mix well. Add ¼ cup peppermint or dehydrated strawberries.

Pour the dark chocolate mixture onto a sheet pan covered in parchment paper and spread into a thin layer. Set in

....

63. Note: We prefer using the 5000 mg/30 ml full-spectrum CBD oil (see appendix) for infusing due to the concentration, which would be 1.4 ml per batch. For lower-concentrated CBD oils, do not use more than 5 ml of oil per batch. Alternately, you can use CBD isolate powder premixed with 5 ml (1 tsp) of canola or fractionated coconut oil. What this means is the stronger the dose of the concentrate, the less you will need to use. You only want to add a small amount of oil so the chocolate will re-harden correctly. Adding too much oil will leave you with soft or sticky chocolate, not hardened. Feel free to change the dosage but be sure to keep the amount of oil you add under 5 ml.

a cooler spot in your workspace, but do not refrigerate. Let the first layer set about 15–20 minutes.

Melt the white chocolate next using a double boiler or in the microwave in 30-second bursts. Stir frequently. Pour the second layer on the first before it is fully hardened so they bind together. Spread across the bottom layer evenly. Top with extra crushed peppermint candies or dehydrated strawberries. Use a sharp knife to score the bark in equal pieces and then tap with any utensil to break apart.

As a chocolate junky, might I add this is also excellent with dried blueberries and lavender buds.

✸ *Chocolate Fudge Truffles*

From Lori Smerz

Serving size: 1 truffle
CBD per serving: 15 mg
Servings per batch: 56
CBD per batch: 840 mg

Ingredients

* ★ 3 cups (18 oz.) semisweet chocolate chips

* ★ 1 can (14 oz.) sweetened condensed milk

* ★ 1 tbs vanilla extract

* ★ 840 mg CBD oil[64]

....

64. Note: We prefer using the 5000 mg/30 ml full-spectrum CBD oil (see appendix) for infusing due to the concentration, which would be 5 ml per batch. Alternately, you can use CBD isolate powder premixed with 5 ml (1 tsp) of canola or fractionated coconut oil.

★ Optional coatings: chocolate sprinkles, Dutch-processed cocoa, ground nuts, chocolate almond bark

In a microwave, melt the chocolate chips with the condensed milk in a glass bowl or a glass pie plate. Melt in 30-second bursts and stir in between. Once melted, stir in the vanilla and the CBD.

Let it set up on the countertop for 30 minutes if you plan to make the truffles right away. Otherwise, you can store in the refrigerator, but remove them 30 minutes ahead of time before scooping into the balls so the chocolate is workable.

With a spoon, scoop enough to fit in the palm of your hand and roll into 1-inch balls. Roll in coating as desired. If you plan to use a coating chocolate, also melt slowly in the microwave 30 seconds at a time, stirring in between. While the coating chocolate is still warm, apply sprinkles or nuts as desired.

Dehydrated Pineapple and Coconut Meditation Munch

From Cheryl Cryer

This sweet and easy natural treat from Cheryl is a perfect snack for those who want something a little sweet without chocolate. I plan to make this for some of my group meditation events.

Serving size: 2 oz.

CBD per serving: 10 mg

Servings per batch: 8

CBD per batch: 80 mg

Ingredients

* ★ 2 cups pineapple, peeled and cut into ½-inch chunks

* ★ ¼ cup maple syrup

* ★ 80 mg CBD oil[65]

* ★ 2 tbs unsweetened coconut, finely shredded

Preheat oven to 175°F. Line a baking sheet with parchment paper and set aside.

In a saucepan on a stove top, simmer the pineapple and maple syrup over medium heat until the pineapple releases its juices—about 5 minutes. Strain and reserve pineapple, returning liquid to saucepan. Simmer until liquid is thick and syrupy, an additional 5 minutes. Add CBD oil, stir thoroughly.

Return pineapple to pan along with coconut and toss gently. Transfer to the parchment-lined baking sheet. Bake for approximately 4 hours, until pineapple is dry and firm.

Remove from oven and cool. Transfer to airtight container and store in a cool location.

❖ Healthy Hemp Granola

From Cheryl Cryer

Serving size: 2 oz.
CBD per serving: 10 mg
Servings per batch: 24
CBD per batch: 240 mg

....

65. Note: We prefer using the 5000 mg/30 ml full-spectrum CBD oil (see appendix) for infusing due to the concentration, which would be 0.5 ml per batch. Alternately, you can use CBD isolate powder.

Ingredients

* ★ 2½ cups mixed raw nuts (we like ½ cup pecans, ¾ cup almonds, 1 cup walnuts)

* ★ ½ cup raw pepitas

* ★ ¼ cup melted coconut oil

* ★ 240 mg CBD oil[66]

* ★ 1 tsp vanilla

* ★ 1 tsp cinnamon

* ★ ¼ cup maple syrup

* ★ Pinch of sea salt

* ★ 1 cup hemp hearts

* ★ 2 tbs chia seeds

* ★ 1 cup unsweetened coconut (shredded or flakes)

* ★ ½ cup pitted and chopped Medjool dates

Preheat oven to 250°F.

Combine raw nuts and pepitas and pulse a few times in a food processor. Be careful not to overprocess, as they should still be chunky pieces. Pour into a bowl and set aside.

....

66. Note: We prefer using the 5000 mg/30 ml full-spectrum CBD oil (see appendix) for infusing due to the concentration, which would be 1.45 ml per batch. For lower-concentrated CBD oils, do not use more than 5 ml of oil per batch. Alternately, you can use CBD isolate powder melted into coconut oil.

In a small bowl, warm the coconut oil in a microwave for just a few seconds until melted. Add CBD oil and blend well. Add vanilla, cinnamon, maple syrup, and sea salt, constantly stirring. Blend in hemp hearts, chia seeds, coconut, and nuts and seed mix from other bowl.

Spread an even layer of the mixture onto two large parchment-lined baking sheets. Bake for 35 minutes, remove from oven.

Add dates into roasted mixture, blend well, and spread back out over pan. Continue to bake for another 30 minutes until granola is a golden brown color.

Remove from oven, cool, and enjoy!

Store in an airtight container.

Juice Shots

Juice shots are becoming increasingly popular, and yet, they are also quite expensive. You can mix up juice shots at home, save money, and add your own CBD oil to them for an extra boost. Remember—juice shots are not made for the taste. They are meant to be downed in one big gulp with a bit of a shock to your system.

Focus Juice Shot

This recipe will help jolt your brain into focus when you are finding yourself easily distracted.

Ingredients

* 1 oz. pure lemon juice
* 1 oz. water

* Up to 2 ml of CBD oil (I use 2 ml of the 1000 mg strength)

* 1 tsp dried turmeric

* Green tree extract (This is available in different forms, such as concentrated in a bottle with a dropper or powdered. You may use a capsule and open it up. Be aware of the number of milligrams you are using and do not exceed 500 milligrams at one time. Green tree extract does contain caffeine.)

* 2 oz. bottle

Pour liquid ingredients (including CBD oil and liquid extract) together first into a 2 oz. bottle and then add the green tree extract (if using a powder) and the turmeric. Shake well and drink in one shot. This can be refrigerated for up to a week.

❀ Relaxing Juice Shot

This juice shot is to help wind you down at the end of a particularly stressful day when the mind needs a bit of peace and your spirit needs to release tension.

Ingredients

* 1 tbs food-grade lavender buds

* ⅛ cup of hot water

* 1 oz. of freshly squeezed blueberry juice (An easy way to do this is with a garlic press instead of using

a juicer. But you can always juice extra and make up a
few bottles at a time.)

* Up to 2 ml of CBD oil (I use 2 ml of the 1000 mg
  strength)

* 2 oz. bottle

Steep the lavender buds in the hot water for 5 minutes
and strain. Allow the lavender water to cool. Add to the 2 oz.
bottle followed by the blueberry juice and CBD oil. Shake
well and drink in one shot. This can be refrigerated for up to
3 days.

CHAPTER 7

The Spirit

We have talked a lot about how CBD can help heal your body and treat several different medical issues and disorders, including fighting pain and inflammation. We have talked about how CBD can help heal your mind and treat several different medical issues that affect the brain, such as with anxiety and depression and other conditions.

Now it's time to focus our attention on spirit.

Building this complete body-mind-spirit connection takes time and work. It doesn't just happen. It's an incredible feeling, and the only way to find it is to work at it. There is no instant gratification choice available.

But how do you get there? How do you start to build the pathways connecting your body-mind-spirit relationship into one cohesively blissful unit? It takes a change in how you do things, why you do things, and sometimes whether or not you do things. This also isn't some type of a one-and-done deal. It is a change of life and learning how to do things differently. Change isn't as difficult as we make it out to be if we break it down into simple steps or tasks. After all, we learned how to do things the way we do; we can learn how to do them a different way too.

You will soon learn this connection doesn't apply only to your CBD use. Once you begin these changes, once you begin feeling these connections, you will want to feel more connections and make more changes.

In this chapter, we will learn different affirmations, meditations, prayers, even rituals, to use in your spiritual practice centered around your CBD use. Learn to celebrate your spirituality, not only at special occasions, but on daily occasions. The events of 2020–2021 gave many of us the opportunity to learn to turn the grind of day-to-day into new positive experiences. It was for many a survival technique, but a technique that can be used even when we aren't amid a pandemic or extreme political upheaval. It is a technique that can help you have a brighter, more positive connection of mind, body, and spirit.

Connecting to Spirit with Meditation

In order to connect to spirit through meditation, you must first learn a little bit about meditation. Meditation is an ancient spiritual practice, which over the years has been altered and branched off into several different types of meditation. While we often hear that meditation is about emptying the mind of all thought, this isn't what it really is at all. Meditation can be different things, but instead of emptying the mind, it is most often about focusing on one thought at a time, recognizing it without judgment, and allowing it to fade into the next thought.

Guided meditations are very helpful for people new to the practice and are plentiful for free throughout the internet. Meditation music (without a guide) is also easy to find and allows your mind to lead you where it may.

Another problem people often have with meditating is visualizing what needs to be visualized. I have learned it is extremely difficult for some people to see things inside of their mind's eye, particularly when it is something they themselves have not experienced in real life. For example, recently I was hosting an online guided meditation session that involved the participants seeing themselves climbing a mountain pass. This may seem easy, until you realize not everyone has seen or walked a mountain pass. It's hard to visualize something that you have not seen before. Preparing ahead of time for a meditation can help you overcome this issue by searching for images online that may help you complete your specific meditation.

When we talk about healing visualizations within the body, this may be difficult for some people to see in their mind's eye. Look up pictures that may help you. Diagrams of chakras, channels, different bodily systems (particularly ones related to any ailments you may have), and photos of cells and organs—whatever it is you need to help you see what your intention is set on.

Meditation preparation may make all the difference in how well the meditation works for you.

Free-flowing meditations can be as specific or as general as you wish. Think about what your intention is and allow it to go from there. Sometimes you may want a quick, easy, refreshing meditation. Other times you may want to go more deeply into meditation to work on healing trauma. What works for you one day may not be what you need on another.

Create Your Setting

To begin your meditation practice, your first step will be to create your setting. Your setting is the environment in which you meditate. While you can meditate anywhere, some places are going to be much easier and more conducive to a good session than others. Can you throw on headphones and listen to a guided meditation on a train while commuting to work? Yes, you can, but it probably won't be your best experience, as it is more difficult to tune out everything when there are distractions all around you.

Creating a special distraction-free location for your meditations can be a part of your spiritual process. Whether you choose a location indoors or out, there are a few tips you will want to keep in mind.

1. Be aware of your lighting situation. Is it too bright? Too dark? Are you at risk for sunburn if sitting in one place too long? If it's too bright, you may end up being distracted, while too dark may find you drifting off to sleep. Keep in mind, though, if this is a nighttime meditation, drifting off to sleep may be a part of your overall goal.

2. Be aware of intruding sounds. Meditating outside is great—unless there is a party close by or road construction, lawn mowers, or other loud noises that would be hard to tune out. Turn off any unnecessary sounds like cell phone ringers and notifications. Noise-cancelling headphones can help make locations more accessible and peaceful.

3. What is the temperature? I honestly don't know which is worse, getting too hot or too cold during a meditation. Both can be distracting. Have a plan to make sure you are comfortable.

4. What posture will you use? Do you plan on sitting or lying down? Be sure to have any necessary cushions, pillows, mats, rolls, bolsters, or any other physical items to ensure your comfort.

5. Add whatever you want to decorate and claim your space. Statues of deities, symbols, crystals and

stones, candles in firesafe containers, incense, and diffusing essential oils all add to your atmosphere.

Setting your mood also includes preparing yourself for meditation. This means getting yourself into the right "set" or frame of mind. You can use CBD to help you do this by first relaxing in a CBD-infused bath. Afterward, use the CBD meditation oil from the last chapter and give yourself a soothing, relaxing massage. If you mixed just the essential oils (and no carrier oil), you can use it on a lit charcoal tablet in a firesafe container or a diffuser to scent the air around you.

Once you have your space planned out, you can move on to the next step: dosing.

Dosing for Meditation

When you take CBD for meditation, you will need to keep in mind that different methods of consumption have different times in which the CBD will take effect. Smoking CBD flower or vaping a CBD concentrate will give you the benefits the fastest. For some people, it is instantaneous; for others, it may take a few minutes to kick in. Using an oil concentrate sublingually (under the tongue) is another fast method, and it generally takes 5–20 minutes to feel the effect. Edibles take the longest to kick in. Of course, everyone has slightly different response times, so you should experiment with different methods to see when you feel the calm and relaxation of CBD come over you.

I often recommend combining methods of consumption for best results. Edibles taken in advance of meditation time have a chance to start working during your meditation. A dose of concentrate oil under my tongue before I sit down helps to relax me more. When I get into position and am ready to go, I can smoke a bowl of CBD flower or take a few hits off of a CBD vape cartridge and then close my eyes.

Combining different methods helps to get a broader range of bioavailability, and it helps keep the endocannabinoid system active, as it is continually catching more CBD in its receptors. This helps intensify the effect and the duration.

The dosage you use for meditation is going to be dependent upon what your normal usage is. If you are already a regular daily user, you will want to increase your dose for meditation time. An easy way to do that is by combining the methods as I mentioned above. Unless you normally use CBD in all these ways throughout the day, then combining different methods is going to give you that extra dose.

If you aren't into smoking or vaping, simply increase the doses of the methods of consumption you do use, but I highly recommend using at least some type of an edible along with an oil concentrate sublingually.

Figuring out what dose works best for you for meditation is going to require a bit of trial and error; unfortunately, that is the downside of CBD—it takes work to find out what works best for you. Start with your normal dosing schedule and then add to it when you want to get ready to meditate. Increase your dosage slowly until you find your perfect place. While trial and error is time consuming, it allows you to get in practice with your meditating too. It also allows for the most personalized and unique dosage plan customized specifically for you.

Getting yourself into the mood is also an important part of meditating. It is more difficult to meditate when you are stressed out or anxious, even though this is when you need meditation the most. Increasing your CBD dosage before meditating helps relieve the stress and anxiety, allowing you to calm yourself and find your focus.

Once you have designed a place for your meditations and learned how to prepare yourself for a meditation practice, it's time to move on and get working.

Breathwork

The beginning of any meditation starts with breathwork designed to help center and ground yourself. Centering can be described as focusing your attention and intention, while grounding deals with the energy you give off and receive.

To begin your breathwork, take a long, deep breath and count as you inhale. Your first couple inhalations, count to four, hold for four counts, and exhale for four counts. As you do this, you will also begin your grounding work. An easy way to ground is to visualize yourself treelike, with roots that reach all the way into the ground. If you are indoors, that is okay—still picture the roots coming out of you and going wherever they need to so they will be able to reach deep into the soil. As they reach into the soil, visualize anything you need to rid yourself of running like tree sap down through your body, through your roots, and into the ground. Bad day at work? Let it run out of you to dissipate into the ground where it can be cleansed and refreshed.

Increase the count on your breathwork to inhale for five counts, hold for five counts, and exhale for five counts. As your breathing slows, see the good, clean, fresh, positive energy from the earth be sucked up into your roots, as if they are drinking in all the good energy they can. This energy flows into your body, replacing the negative energy you dispelled.

If it is comfortable for you, go ahead and slow your breathing even more to a six-count cycle. Continue visualizing the energy exchange until you feel relaxed and ready to move on with the main event of your meditation session.

Listening to the Body Meditations

Spending meditative time checking in with your body is essential. Think of these meditations as a phone call to check in and see how things are going. It's your first step in communication. No meditations, no phone call, no communication.

If you do not normally meditate, no problem. I have often heard people say they cannot meditate because they cannot empty their minds, and I believed this for years.

But what I thought about meditation was wrong. Meditation isn't about emptying your mind of all thoughts; it's about focusing and directing your thoughts to a specific point. In this case, we will be focusing on and directing our thoughts to different areas of the body. If other thoughts enter your mind while doing these practices, that is okay. Recognize distractions, acknowledge them, and file them away to deal with later if necessary. Then move on. Meditation doesn't have to be a perfect, uninterrupted, 100-percent-focused session. What is perfect is often imperfection and whatever works for you.

✿ Drop-In Relaxing Body Scan

Throughout your day, particularly if you are in a stressed mode, take a moment for a quick drop-in body scan meditation. You can do this meditation anywhere you have a moment to sit by yourself and close your eyes for a few minutes. It's perfect for a quick pick-me-up, particularly with a fast-acting dose of CBD. (A fast-acting dose includes smoking, vaping, or a concentrated oil under the tongue.)

Take three deep breaths in and out through your nose. Allow your breath to return to its normal rate and focus on the rise and fall of your chest for a few moments.

If you can do this meditation without shoes on, take a moment to stretch your toes and wiggle them around. Arch and flex your feet and rotate your ankles. Wiggle your fingers, stretch them out, rotate your wrists. Tilt your head to each side, and then let it circle around in both directions. Lift your shoulders up toward your ears for a moment, hold, and then relax.

Does anything feel off to you? Are any muscles too tight, cramped, or kinked? Send soothing thoughts to any parts of your body that need it. Visualize healing energy flowing to any place your body needs it. You may want to see it as a white or green healing light. Focus it wherever it needs to go. Allow your body to relax where need be. Don't be afraid to use your hands to massage tight areas. You can remain in your meditative state and still move a bit.

Your emotional body is as important as your physical body. What is on your mind? What is in your heart? Are you stressed, confused, sad, overwhelmed? Release any negativity you may have picked up during the day. Acknowledge the feeling is there, without judgment, and allow it to pass. For the moment, set it aside to deal with later. For now, relax, and let go.

For a few more breaths, bring to mind a favorite scene and place yourself in it. It may be a real or imaginary place, as long as it is a place that makes you feel happy, relaxed, or even blessed.

When you are ready, take another deep breath, let it out slowly, and reopen your eyes. This quick pick-me-up meditation may be just the thing you need to get through difficult days. Remember, meditation isn't a chore; it's far more of a blessing that we often need to remind ourselves we are entitled to. Taking a break from a hectic, painful day to check in, refocus, and reevaluate is the perfect example of proactive self-care.

✸ *Morning Check-In Meditation*

When you wake in the morning, position yourself comfortably on your back and re-close your eyes. Take a few deep breaths, shaking off any grogginess, yawning away the last remnants of sleep. Take a moment to feel your position in the bed. Feel where your body meets the mattress below you. Feel any sheets, blankets, clothing lying on top of you. Notice the outer feelings against your skin and body. Is the air warm or cool on your face? There is no pressure. No rush. Just simply feeling the things in contact with your physical body.

Once you finish feeling the outer connections, turn your focus inward. Start gently telling your body it's time to wake up. Send positive energy to each part of your body as you work with it.

Stretch out your face muscles. Scrunch up your eyes and hold them tightly closed before letting them relax but remain closed. Move your tongue around in your mouth. Over and around your teeth. Open your mouth really wide for a moment, stretching it all out. Stretch your lips to the sides in a big, wide-open grin. Then pucker them up into a tight-lipped smooch before relaxing once again.

How do you feel so far? Truly feel your body with each of these movements. Check in and ensure everything feels like it should. Note any pain you find as you go and evaluate it. Is it discomfort? Something more serious? Is this "normal" for you? Is there anything different about it?

Next, move your attention to your neck. Stretch it out by pulling your chin into the air. Turn your head to the left and then to the right, holding it for a moment in each direction. Tilt your head left and right, holding each position. Roll your shoulders back, gently scrunching them into the bed. Reverse direction and roll them forward. Send positive energy, waking up the muscles. Imagine the warmth of sunlight washing over you as you awaken more and more of your body.

Try to feel inside the very nerves and muscles that allow you to move. Picture in your mind the muscles working in unison, the electric impulses from the brain traveling down pathways telling the body what to do. Envision it as you move about.

Continue to direct your focus internally to each of these movements. Work on isolating the sensations of the individual muscles that work together to complete these physical tasks. Feel each muscle as it stretches and relaxes.

From your shoulders, pick one arm to wake up and work your way down to the fingers. Bend and straighten the arm at the elbow. Move to the wrist and circle it in both directions. Always focusing. Always sensing and feeling each movement. Wiggle your fingers in a low-key jazz hand. Stretch the fingers as far away from each other as you can. Ball them into a tight fist and then relax. Each movement a sensation all its own. When you finish with one arm, continue with the other.

After your arms, let's move to your torso. Tighten the muscles in your chest. It is hard for many people to isolate these muscles, particularly older women, but work at it and you will find them. Finding these muscles is the first step in learning to connect and listen to them. Next, isolate and tighten your stomach muscles. Hold for a moment and then relax. Tighten all the muscles of your lower abdomen, including your derriere. Hold and release. Wake up your body with a smile. Let it know you are ready to start your day and look forward to it.

Move to your legs. Choose one leg to work with first, bending your knee while keeping your foot flat on the bed. Let your knee fall to the outside to stretch out your hip joint. Center your attention on the hip joint and then the knee joint. Pull your knee back up and lift your leg into the air as high or as low as is comfortable for you, but enough to give you a slight stretch in the leg. Switch to the other leg and repeat these movements.

Twirl your feet both left and right, working your ankle joints. Feel for any friction. Listen for popping. Point your toes and stretch, followed by a flex and hold. Stretch your toes apart as far as you can and then close them down tightly before relaxing once again.

Where did you find any issues? Anything your body wants you to know today? Spend as much time as you need feeling your way around inside your body, connecting to muscles, joints, and even organs. Focus is key, but it will take practice. Learn to listen to what your body is telling you.

Once you are ready, take a few more deep breaths, and then open your eyes, ready for the day.

✸ Bedtime Check-In Meditation

Like the Morning Check-In meditation, this is going to occur while you are in bed, but this time once you are ready to head off to la-la land.

At the end of the day, it may be exceedingly difficult for some people to wind down. The thoughts of the day may be darting around in your head. Plans for the next day may be anticipated. Many of us have a hard time shutting our thinking process down at the end of the day, making it difficult to get a good night's sleep. This meditation not only helps create the body-mind-spirit connection, but it also allows you something neutral to focus on before drifting off to sleep. It is a way to disengage your brain from the outer world and focus instead on your inner self. This helps many people fall asleep easier, as they have purposely directed their focus from outer activity to the inner activity of the body. This is soothing.

Thoughts no longer compete for your attention because your attention is already absorbed elsewhere: on you.

When you are ready to fall asleep, lie on your back in a comfortable position. Feel where your body meets the mattress. Notice any sheets, blankets, clothing lying on top of you. Acknowledge the outer feelings against your skin and body.

You will be singling each body part out and tightening it up for a few moments and then releasing it, letting go of any tension left from the day. Let your body know it is time to relax and rest. Thank it for working hard and taking care of you throughout the day. Remember, as energy beings, our bodies are our shells. They are what protect us and keep us alive. We need to be mindful of and take care of our bodies and protect them in return. When we are out of touch with our bodies, we take them for granted and expect them to function all the time. When we connect with our bodies, we care for them. We honor them. We protect them. We understand the body needs care, rest, and love just as much as it needs food and water. When our bodies function at their best, our brains and spirit can function at their best. When we are sluggish, uncomfortable, and down, it reflects in our bodies performing poorly. Let your body know you appreciate the hard work it does for you every day.

Start gently telling your body it's time to relax and go to sleep. Send positive energy to each part of your body as you work with it.

Stretch out your face muscles. Scrunch up your eyes and hold them tightly closed before letting them relax but remaining closed. Move your tongue around in your mouth. Over and around your teeth. Open your mouth really wide for a moment, stretching it all out. Stretch your lips to the sides in a big, wide-open grin. Then pucker them up into a tight-lipped smooch before relaxing once again.

How do you feel so far? Truly feel your body with each of these movements. Check in and ensure everything feels like it should. Note any pain you find as you go and evaluate it. Is it discomfort? Something more serious? Is this "normal" for you? Is there anything different about it?

Next, move your attention to your neck. Stretch it out by pulling your chin into the air. Turn your head to the left and then to the right, holding it for a moment in each direction. Tilt your head left and right, holding each position. Roll your shoulders back, gently scrunching them into the bed. Reverse direction and roll them forward. Send positive energy, relaxing each area of your body.

Continue to direct your focus internally to each of the movements you make. Work on isolating the sensations of the individual muscles that work together to complete these physical tasks. Feel each muscle as it stretches and relaxes.

From your shoulders, pick one arm to focus on and work your way down to the fingers. Bend and straighten the arm at the elbow. Move to the wrist and circle it in both directions. Always focusing. Always sensing and feeling each movement.

Wiggle your fingers in a low-key jazz hand. Stretch the fingers as far away from each other as you can. Ball them into a tight fist and then relax. Each movement a sensation all its own. When you finish with one arm, continue with the other.

Honor each part of your body as you acknowledge the work it did for the day. Be thankful and appreciative of how your body works. Let your body know it's time to wind down and get some well-earned rest.

After your arms, let's move to your torso. Tighten the muscles in your chest. It is hard for many people to isolate these muscles, particularly older women, but work at it and you will find them. Finding these muscles is the first step in learning to connect and listen to them. Next, isolate and tighten your stomach muscles. Hold for a moment and then relax. Tighten all the muscles of your lower abdomen, including your derriere. Hold and release.

Move to your legs. Choose one leg to work with first, bending your knee while keeping your foot flat on the bed. Let your knee fall to the outside to stretch out your hip joint. Center your attention on the hip joint and then the knee joint. Pull your knee back up and lift your leg into the air as high or as low as is comfortable for you, but enough to give you a slight stretch in the leg. Switch to the other leg and repeat these movements.

Twirl your feet both left and right, working your ankle joints. Feel for any friction. Listen for popping. Point your toes and stretch, followed by a flex and hold. Stretch your toes apart as far as you can and then close them down tightly before relaxing once again.

Envision the muscles relaxing, resting. See joints as they lie in place, motionless. Ready for respite. The electrical impulses from the brain slow in a dimmer light. Rest is at hand as the body goes into sleep mode. You will be refreshed and recharged in the morning, but for now, keep those eyes closed and drift off to sleep.

Checking in with your body can be done at any time of the day, whether you do every morning and every night or not. There are some times when you really need to far more often than others—after an injury or surgery or during a serious illness. COVID-19 has shown us how fast a medical condition can turn on you. If you feel the need to sit down in the middle of the day and do a quick check-in with your body, do it. If it's trying to get your attention because there is a potential problem, you don't want to ignore it.

Body scan meditations are excellent for daily practice of your visualization skills. Working with them frequently will help you build your skills for other specialized, advanced meditations.

Increase Your Meditation Repertoire

Use your improved visualization skills to add more in-depth meditations to your practice. These workings will help you learn how to connect your energy to outside sources and bring those energies into your body.

✻ *Light It Up Connection Meditation*

One of the great benefits of CBD is it works where our body needs it to. The endocannabinoid system, being responsible for keeping our other biological systems in balance, knows what your body needs. CBD helps the ECS to work more efficiently while in overdrive. It knows you on the inside, which is part of what makes this connection meditation fun. When you are ready, begin by holding your CBD product in your hand in a clear glass container. Turn the container over in your hands several times, allowing the contents to mix where possible. Visualize energy as a green light at your fingertips as you make these rotations. Not an overpowering energy, but a glowing light, slowly streaming out of your fingertips and through the glass, snaking its way into your product—swirling, climbing, eventually coating or combining and becoming absorbed. Let the energy communicate to the product what you need most. Focus on the healing energies you are seeking. Allow the glowing light energy to deliver your message to your product. We know cannabinoids will go where needed. Visualizing the connection from you to the product, which will then come back to you again, completes a circle.

✻ *The Spirit of Cannabis Meditation*

Many different spiritual traditions believe that all plants have a spirit or soul of their own. The cannabis plant is no exception, with the spirit of cannabis being different in different traditions. The spirit of cannabis helps you to build the body-mind-spirit connection. Whether you are using a THC-rich strain or one with none but rich in CBD, the spirit of cannabis entwines with your spirit to help make the connection complete. Think back to when we learned about the endocannabinoid system. When CBD or THC attaches to the CB1 and CB2 receptors, they are completing a unit. When this unit is completed, the body can do what it needs to do better. The cannabinoids in the cannabis plant are designed to work specifically with these receptors, showing cannabis was meant to work with us, not against us as politicians and the rich have made it. The spirit of cannabis works the same way with our spirit as the cannabinoids work with our receptors. When they entwine together, the spirit can do what it needs to do better.

Cannabis is a generously giving plant. It gives everything of itself to provide for us physically, mentally, and spiritually. When it dies, we are able to benefit incredibly from its use in many ways. When you start to think about it this way, it's hard not to make a spiritual connection. This meditation will help you make your own connection to the spirit of cannabis.

Either sit or lie down in a comfortable position. Slow your breathing to a deep yet comfortable pace for you. Focus on your breathing. Remember, meditation isn't clearing your mind, it's focusing it. Right now, spend a few minutes focusing on your breathing until you feel calm and relaxed and ready to move on.

When you are set, begin by visualizing a small, bright green light in front of you. Floating. Drifting gently. It sends out bright, happy, healthy vibrations, reverberating from its core. The light begins to grow. As it grows bigger, it also grows brighter. As you look deep into the light, you see swirls of darker green dancing, gliding through the light. They begin to collide in waves, conjoining. Taking shape. Pay attention to the shape that begins forming in front of you, for it is the shape of spirit. This is the spirit of the plant.

The inky waves crash together, forming delicate tendrils. The tendrils, like wisps of smoke, float in the air, but instead of dissipating, they grow. They grow stronger, longer, bolder, more defined. As the tendrils circle around each other, they grow into stems, yet maintain their darker, inky green shadow. You watch as several stems in front of you grow at an accelerated rate. Buds quickly form, then uncoil into giant cannabis fan leaves. The fan leaves grow incredibly large, surrounded by the bright green light, emanating a healthy green glow. The area in front of you is covered in the leaves. They stop growing but continue to sway in the air, momentarily, calmly, before shifting and swirling into a spiral of leaves of green light until they begin taking another form. The figure begins to take shape in front of you. The bright green light softens and fades, revealing the spirit fully to you.

How does the spirit appear to you? Take in their features, their mannerisms, their aura. Look into their eyes. What is their name? Sense their energy with yours.

When you are ready, visualize your own spirit reaching out to your new friend. The light of their green aura brightens as you reach for them, gently swirling as it reaches out toward you too. As your two spirits meet, their green light spirals throughout your energy field, leaving a trail, scattering itself as it travels. The spirit gives of themself, sharing their bounty, a smile upon their face. They look up into your eyes one last time, waiting, watching, as the last of their energy is absorbed by your spirit. They nod and fade into the bright green light. As it breaks, it clouds and disperses.

Visualizing the spirit for yourself is another step in completing your own body-mind-spirit connection. It also helps to build reverence and respect for what the plant can do for you.

✺ Healing Meditation

This healing meditation is particularly good for those who have a more difficult time visualizing with their mind's eye. For those who have visualization issues, this may make it easier for you, and it also shows you how you can break down meditations into aspects you are familiar with instead of struggling with ones you aren't. This is a main key to meditation. You do not have to worry about your image being 100 percent correct; you only have to understand what your image represents. If you need to, look up some diagrams or images that deal with your ailment and how it affects your body; do so ahead of time to help you out with the process. For example, one of the ailments I use CBD for the most is my arthritis. My hip and knee joints in particular need all kinds of extra help. I have seen plenty of X-rays and MRIs of these joints to be able to picture them in my mind quite easily.

I also use CBD to help with my anxiety. This is a bit more difficult to visualize, but I know that the process of calming my anxiety happens inside my brain. I can imagine the cells, pathways, and chemicals in my brain in any way I want to if I understand that what I am visualizing represents those cells, pathways, and chemicals. The pictures in your eye do not have to exactly match reality as long as you understand what the pictures represent.

Get yourself into a comfortable position, and as you take a dose of your CBD, close your eyes and visualize the path the CBD takes. This may be through your digestive system or through your respiratory system depending on what consumption method you use.

Picture what you have consumed in a way that is easy for you. Maybe the CBD is a certain color as it travels throughout your body. Perhaps you see it as a vehicle driving or flying where it needs to go carrying a horde of little workers who are there to do repair work. You can picture it any way you want to, which makes it easy for you to envision the CBD traveling throughout your body to the area where the work needs to be done.

Once it makes it to where it needs to be, visualize the CBD working to repair your ailment. See it in a way that makes sense to you, whether you need to see it as a glowing-colored light or perhaps a crew of mini worker droids flying in for repairs. It's your meditation—you can visualize what you need to any way you want. You do not have to try to imagine what it looks like when CB1 and CB2 receptors attract CBD molecules and send chemical messages to the brain, which then, in turn, sends other messages through electrical impulses or other chemical releases. Use what you know and see the repair process take place in a way that makes sense for you—a way that is easily visualized. Witness the healing taking place.

One of the ways I use this meditation is when my sciatica acts up. I visualize the CBD going straight to the joints that are in shooting pain. Once it is there, I envision the CBD turning to a cooling blue light. My sciatica burns terribly, so a cooling blue light helps my brain counteract the burning sensation in my back. As the CBD works on the pain, I use my visualization to help focus my attention on cooling the joints down. While green is usually associated with healing, I have found for this ailment, blue works best for me. Focus your attention and your intention on where it is needed to speed up your own healing process. Experiment with different scenarios to see how they differ and what works for you.

Connecting to Spirit in the Kitchen

As a society, we have become extremely detached from our food and where it comes from. Pushes for localized sourcing and sustainable practices are beginning to gain more traction, and when this happens, we begin to learn more about our food supply chain. Learning about the food supply chain is an important part of your spiritual practice. Honestly. Think about it. It is difficult to make a complete mind-body-spirit connection if your mind has no idea what you are putting into your body. I am not going to tell you that means you need to eat a certain way; I will leave those choices completely up to you. However, whatever those choices are, still do the research into where your food comes from and what it contains. For some people, learning these things does end up changing their normal diet. What works for you works for you, but be aware of what your food is and where it comes from. Knowing what you are working with is essential to obtain your desired results. To make the connection complete, information must be obtained to achieve wisdom.

The kitchen witch part of my eclectic path loves to infuse my energy and intentions into recipes when preparing them. This goes hand in hand with knowing where your food comes from. If you prepare your own meals with fresh ingredients, it is a much more personal, spiritual experience. You are spending time and energy with these ingredients. Treat them with loving respect, as they will provide you with nourishment.

This transfers over to creating your own CBD products. When you work with the different ingredients, you infuse your energy into them. We learned earlier when it comes to CBD, it is extremely important to know the source of your flower or the concentrates you are using. Ensure quality by caring enough to do your research so when you infuse your own energy into your concoctions, it's not going to waste on something of poor quality.

Blessing the CBD Flower

When working with flower, I like to do a bit of a blessing on the plant material itself before starting any of my processes—so before decarboxylating. There are different ones you can do, so I am going to include a few different ways you can bless your flower. Affirmations and blessings don't have to be a big production. In fact, it's the little things you do that quickly become habit. It's much easier to make changes when they are small. Sprinkling in a phrase or rhyme here and there, stirring in an intention or blessing—these little things build together to create perfect connections.

Dried flower can be sticky, and you don't want to mix the oils from your skin with it, so to keep it pure and free from contamination, don't touch it any more than you have to. This hands-off approach helps create a bit of a reverence for it. I prefer to use wooden utensils when possible with mine and avoid plastic as much as possible. I store it in glass containers. Some people will use gloves when handling it; I personally do not, but it is up to you. For the small amount I do touch it, I would rather have the physical connection to the plant than have a plastic barrier between. Again, it's all about building the connection.

When I purchase flower, the first thing I do is remove it from its packaging and place it in a glass container. I have some great ones with airtight lids painted with a mandala on top. These clear jars allow me to have a good view of the flower. It allows for things like moonbeams to have a good view of the flower too.

✿ Full Moon Blessing

If you live in a place where it would be safe to do so, place your flower (or concentrated oils) in a clear (colored is okay if it is still translucent) glass container outside under the full moon. If it isn't ideal to leave things outside overnight, place them in front of a window where the moon's energy can reach out to it. (If you happen to smoke flower from a bong or bubbler, you can make moon water to use by placing it in a glass container in the moonlight too for a little bit of extra magic!) When you place the container, project positive healing energies toward it and say under the moon:

> *Moon above, full and bright*
> *Send your energy,*
> *Through your light.*
> *Shine down through the night*
> *Enrich this [flower, oil, or water]*
> *For my might.*
> *Thank you.*

Take a moment to visualize blue-white light beams reaching down from the moon into the glass to imbue the strength and magic of the moon. Leave it overnight, and in the morning, once it has been moon blessed, be sure to store it in a place out of direct sunlight until ready to use. You can look up the correspondences for each month's moon, too, if you are looking for a specific type of energy or blessing.

Connecting with Spirit in the Garden

Combine the four elements together by throwing some seeds in dirt (earth), adding some water (water), a bit of light in the perfect amount (fire), and some carbon dioxide (air), and poof—magic—a plant that helps bring your body into perfect balance.

If you are able to grow your own flower, you already have an incredible connection to it. You nurture the buds from the time they are a tiny little seed. Growing indoors on a small scale isn't easy, and it can require special lighting, heating, and cooling for the plants in order to achieve a successful crop. If you are growing for THC, certain conditions must be met for plants to thrive, and they must be watched to harvest at just the right time. The plants count on you to meet their needs, and in return you count on the plant to meet yours. It's a beautiful relationship, and there is no reason why you cannot treat it as such.

❀ Blessing the Seeds

Next time you are ready to start your seeds, hold them in the palm of your dominant hand. Cup your other hand over them. As you hold them, think about the massive energy these seeds contain. They will grow from these tiny seeds into plants several feet tall with bunches of leaves and flowers all over them. Can you feel the energy in these seeds waiting to burst forth? Envision the process the seed goes through, from splitting and forming into a little sprout to growing those first cotyledons to full-budded colas with rich little trichomes. What an incredible process. Thank the seeds. Think about it, and then honestly thank the seeds. They are going to go through all this change and growth for your benefit in the end. While you put in effort and other essentials, it is the plant that gives its whole life—all the energy it has transformed and stored in the buds will be removed and transformed again when the cannabinoids work with your endocannabinoid system. This process of transformation is at the heart of energy workings. Thank and bless these seeds in whatever way suits you best. Send them energy. Thank them. Talk to them if you want. Build the relationship.

Creating a Spiritual Connection

Creating and crafting in the kitchen includes everything from decarbing flower to mixing up a smoothie. Anything you do in preparation for your meals, beverages, oils, and other products can be done with specific intentions added into the process. Each of these additions works on building the relationship and increasing the spiritual connections. Let me give you an example.

When I am making a citrus smoothie blast, this recipe requires several steps. As I zest the peels, I focus on what the zest contributes to the overall recipe: it brightens it up with a powerful dose of limonene, a terpene that has the benefits of being uplifting and cleansing. Just the smell alone puts you in a good mood with its cheery nature. It has the same effect once it is in your body. As I take off the rest of the peels, I think about how I will dry and preserve them with their energy to grind up for later use in other ways, such as in teas. When I make the juice, I focus on the process of the nutrients being removed from the pulp. The things we don't need can be set aside to focus on those we do.

When I combine all the ingredients together in the blender, I can focus on different aspects depending on what I need each day. Sometimes I might focus on the cow that produced the milk that was processed into the yogurt that will now nourish me. When preparing and consuming food items, I often focus on it going where I need it to go. I might think about the people who picked the fruit I have juiced. Following the food path backward is one type of connection; it traces the energy conversions many times over. Recognizing and acknowledging your place in this line can be a humbling experience. If I'm in a particularly down mood, I may focus on the refreshing citrus scent as it blends together.

If life is a bit chaotic, I may focus on that notion—sometimes turmoil (like a blender) can create something wonderful (like an awesome smoothie). Each of these small ideas brings with it positive intentions.

You can infuse your work with your energy and intentions. Tasks such as slicing, dicing, and chopping are rhythmic and make it easy to focus on infusing your work with whatever intention you need. Choose a word or two you can chant either aloud or silently in your mind. For example, you can focus on good health, and as you work, repeat over and over "good health." See yourself as the representation of what good health means to you.

Blending and stirring with a spoon or spatula is a great way to infuse your work with your energy. Again, you may take a rhythmic approach and chant to build energy to instill in your product. Make up your own song or just plainly state your need. What works for you is what works for you. Focus on the intention you want to send, and most importantly, let yourself send it. Feel and see the energy traveling from you through your arm into the utensil you are using and then disperse into the ingredients you are working with.

Raising Energy

Where does energy come from? It is up to you: You can pull the energy up through your feet from the earth below you, or you can pull it down from the sky above you. You can begin seeing it in the location of your mind, your heart, or one of your chakra areas. Where do you want to pull it from? What feels right to you? If one of your chakra areas is blocked and is manifesting in a medical issue, you can see how this connection can be helpful. For example, if I have endometriosis, a condition associated with the root chakra, I can send energy from my root chakra to the medicine I am preparing to help treat the pain. My root chakra is reaching out saying, "Hey! Look over here. This is where you are going to need to help. This is where the problem is." This universal energetic connection helps prepare my medicine for exactly what I need it to do. It may sound a bit crazy; I completely understand. It wasn't until it really started working for me and my own connection started building that I became a believer myself. The easiest way to become a believer is to try it. And if it doesn't work for you, then you haven't lost anything either.

Personally, my favorite method for raising energy is dancing. Singing and dancing around the kitchen while I work builds the energy that I can then release into my workings or whatever it is I am preparing. It also helps me get my steps in for the day, so a complete win-win.

It is so important to remember, if you make your spiritual practice something *you* will enjoy, then you will practice.

Follow Your Instincts

If someone tells you to do something a certain way in your practice and it doesn't feel right to you, don't do it. Your practice isn't about you being uncomfortable. Yes, there are times we need to face things we don't want to, but those aren't the things I am talking about here. I am talking about when you feel strongly about something and you feel it is wrong for you. Follow your gut. When your intuition is trying to tell you something, you need to listen to it. Do the things that make you happy and feel good. Do the hard work when you need to, but make your spiritual practice personalized to you.

If your practice isn't enjoyable to you, you won't want to do it anyway. Why would you? But if you aren't enjoying it, that simply means that whatever it is you are doing isn't right for you—no matter if someone told you it should be. If you don't like to be hot and sticky, hot yoga probably won't be your thing even if all your friends love it. The idea of dancing around your kitchen to '80s music might make you cringe. Maybe you prefer music from the 2010 decade? Maybe you would like to go running around the block to build energy? Maybe you like to drum. Or sing opera. Or kickbox. Or have sex. How do you like to raise energy? What works for you? Whatever it is, that is what you use. Don't feel guilty if you don't feel what others say you should. So, one last time, if no one has ever told you before, you really do have permission to find your spirituality where you need to. Follow your own path and don't be afraid to travel it alone. It is when you are by yourself you find your true self.

Making the Mundane Spiritual

There are other ways to help build your spiritual connection in the kitchen, including the equipment you use and how you use it. I prefer to use as many natural products—wood and glass—over plastic as much as possible: wood spoons, glass measuring cups and bowls, wood cutting boards. While it isn't realistic to avoid all unnatural products, I simply like to eliminate them where I can and keep my workings as natural and in line with the elements as possible. I do like to have some things that are not used for any type of mundane purpose, such as my mortar and pestle, moon water bottles, and certain containers and spoons. While this may not be something you normally think about, go ahead—think about it. Choose a few specific pieces for yourself. They don't have to be expensive, but you can personalize these choices any way you want. You can do whatever you want. Let me say that again: You can do whatever you want.

Create Intention and Affirmations

I know a lot of times people want to be told specific words to say when setting intentions and affirmations, and because I know you want them, I am going to give them to you. But I am also going to give you this advice: This is your starting point, not your ending point. Don't let someone else's words always speak for you. It's okay to get a jump start. It's okay to brainstorm. But when it comes right down to it, you know you better than anyone else does, and your goal here is to get to know yourself even better. My words can only help you to a certain point. After that, it is up to you. Find the words your soul wants to use. But I do completely understand how awesome it is to have a guidebook and map in hand before setting out to explore the world in front of you.

One of my favorite ways to infuse and set intentions is simply by singing whatever comes into my head at the time. It doesn't have to rhyme, though sometimes it does. I often can't remember it moments later even though I just said it. There is often no discernable tune, but sometimes I will sing to the tune of a well-known song like "Row, Row, Row Your Boat." I might sing loud; I might sing soft. One thing I never do is sing well, because I simply can't. But that doesn't stop me. Why should it? I'm not singing for anyone's approval. I am singing because that is what my spirit wants to be doing. It wants to happily express itself in (sometimes downright silly) song. And so, I let it. You can let your spirit do things that others may deem silly. We're allowed, and your spirit will appreciate the chance at something lighthearted. While setting intention is indeed serious business that we need to do with respect, we can also do it with a little fun. Having fun doesn't mean we aren't committed or serious. It means we are enjoying the work we are doing.

Let's go ahead and get you some starting points for affirmations and chants.

Cheers to Good Health

One of the most often-used intentions is for good health. It's the main reason we use CBD, so it makes perfect sense most of us will have either good health (physical, mental, emotional) or healing in mind. Some people use these terms interchangeably, others do not, stating, "good health" is more focused on maintaining an already achieved level of health while healing is for overcoming an ailment. It is up to you how you see it. You know your own intention better than others. But since you are using these as a starting point, you can easily rework something if you need it to fit just a little bit better. Personally, the way I see it is we are always striving for good health, and life itself is a continual healing process. We are always trying to heal ourselves from something. With the damage we have done to ourselves from an environmental standpoint alone, the damage is never fully healed. The goal is to be able to fully heal ourselves spiritually before the ability to heal ourselves physically runs out (we die). If you ask me, that's why we are here. I have been incredibly surprised over the past several years how my relationship with a plant has helped me to grow. (No pun intended—this time, anyway.)

✺ Affirmations for Good Health and Healing

Remember, you can use these as starting points for you to find your own words. Try them until what you need comes to you. Alter them as you need to make them fit your situation and the task you are performing. Speak them, chant them, sing them, and dance around if you want. Build more energy. It is entirely up to you. I do like to work with a lot of rhymes when doing certain tasks, particularly things like stirring or chopping, which can be done rhythmically and incorporated into performing the affirmation as a chant with its own percussion. As always, you do you.

When we refer to "healing" in these affirmations, it refers to whatever type of healing you need. For example, if your focus is on controlling arthritis, you want to focus your intentions on your working being filled with anti-inflammatory properties. You want to envision the swelling going down in joints or other affected parts of the body. If your focus is on a more generic "good health" type of vibe—maybe you are in great shape and are working more at maintaining than healing—you can focus on the way your good health makes you feel. Focus on energy. Vibrancy.

Remember, some days are bad days, and on those bad days, anything we can muster is better than nothing at all. Even on the darkest days, we can still look for a silver lining. We also need to always be honest with ourselves if we are going to truly know ourselves, so when you feel old or down or falling apart, admit to it. Admitting how we feel is the first step to changing how we feel. Denying how we feel doesn't help us stop feeling that way; in fact, it keeps us in the slump, and the slump is not where we want to be.

Tailor your thoughts to meet your needs to infuse your energy's intention.

Empower this [oil/plant/mixture/recipe] with my intention: good health, healing, and illness prevention.

Instill this [oil/plant/mixture/recipe] with healing strength; tune us to the same wavelength.

Bless my working as I go. My energy I share, to and fro. Complete the circle, plant to me, when I use it, shall it be.

As I [stir, chop, slice], these words I say, strengthen my work, this is the way. (Any *Mandalorian* fans out there? Inspiration can come from all kinds of places!)

Truth be told, I feel old. Imbue I do, to feel new.

This work I do, will refresh and renew.

My love inside, I do share, to health and wellness, for those I care. (When sharing whatever you are preparing with others.)

While of course you don't have to, expressing intention verbally makes it stronger. When you say something out loud, it makes it more real. It gives it more power. You are engaging more of your senses, more of yourself into your working. Let yourself use all the power you have available to you.

❀ Affirmations for Promoting Calmness

When anxiety hits, it may help to use affirmations to help relax and calm your mind. You can use these affirmations either while you are preparing recipes (and send your intentions to your working) or when you are medicating, particularly if you are having an anxiety flare.

I am calm. I am at peace. I am well.

I am cool. I am calm. I am collected.

I am capable and can care for myself.

I am safe. I am protected. I am okay.

I am guided by spirit. I am at peace.

I release that which I cannot control. I relax, and I let go.

Anxiety does not choose for me. I choose for me.

Your CBD is always going to work best when you put your mind and spirit in line with the healing you need from your medicine. Put your positive energy into your medicine, and your medicine will be filled with positive energy—a great thing for when you really need it!

The same is also true if you are in a bad mood and doing prep work. Guess what? You are putting your negative energy into what you are doing. It is important to remember both ways are true, so if you are going to give off either good vibes or bad ones, you may as well choose for them to be good ones. This being said, your prep work should be a happy time, not feel like a chore. When things are no longer enjoyable, we stop doing them. Do your prep work when you are happy and in a good mood. It is hard not to enjoy the work once you start doing it. Blending herbs together on a sunny day, there isn't much that is better.

Always be conscious of what you send out to your work and to others. Be conscious of what they send out to you.

If you notice certain people trigger your anxiety, it's time to look into why and do something about it. Healing is about confronting and facing what we must in order to repair damage done. When you are ready to fully heal, you will know.

The Power of Prayer

Whether you work with a deity or some other form of higher power, you are most likely familiar with the power of prayer. While some people see prayer as a direct request or communication to a deity, others see it as sending a message to the universe at large. Prayer is asking for a transformation of energy for a specific outcome; in this way, it is very similar to the concept of a spell.

Your CBD-related prayers may include asking your deities or other higher power to bless your CBD, whether it is in an oil, tincture, flower, or other form. Just as when people sit down to give thanks and ask for a blessing for food, you may sit down and ask for a blessing on your CBD. When it comes right down to it, CBD is a natural medicine given to us by our creator to work in conjunction with our endocannabinoid system. It is a gift to help us heal, and for that, some may feel it is appropriate to offer up prayers of thankfulness.

Whomever you send your prayers to is up to you. Personally, when it comes to any sort of cannabis, I work with several different deities. Sometimes it is Ganesh, the overcomer of obstacles. During my cancer treatments, I worked with him intensely. He is also a god of ganja. Other times I may send up prayers of thanks to the Green Man, Pan, or Bloudewedd, all of whom I associate with cannabis due to their distinct ties to nature.

These are short prayers you can use to ask for a blessing upon your CBD product, followed by more short prayers of thankfulness. Feel free to mix and match them up to combine into different prayers to suit your needs. Begin and end your prayer with what greeting and closing work best for you.

✹ Prayers Requesting Blessings

Bless this plant, which you have provided upon our green earth.

Let the nourishment it received through air, fire, water, and earth now come to nourish me.

Bless us both as we two become one.

★

I ask for your blessings upon this [CBD/flower].

Guide it to enrich my health physically, mentally, emotionally, and spiritually.

By your will and nature's grace, I accept your blessings.

★

Blessed be this which I take into me.

Blessed be this which aids me.

Blessed be this which heals me.

Blessed be this which nurtures me.

★

Grant this [CBD/flower] your healing strength.

Direct it to where it may have the greatest benefit.

Heal my self, body, spirit, and mind.

★

Bless this [CBD/flower] with your might and love.

Sharing with me your strength and care.

Your blessings help me to fight [whatever your ailment is].

Your blessings help me to live.

✿ Prayers of Thankfulness

Thank you for providing the means to help heal my body.

The healing you help to provide allows me to live a more whole, complete life.

★

I give thanks for the CBD you have provided.

I give thanks for the plant and the knowledge to use it.

I give thanks for the healing it provides for my body and mind.

★

I am grateful and thankful for all the benefits CBD has provided.

I am grateful for the way it eases my pain.

I am thankful for the way it eases my mind.

I am grateful and thankful for the relief and calm it brings me.

*

I give my gratitude for the blessings provided by CBD and the cannabis plant.

I give my gratitude for the completeness it brings to me, filling in gaps to make me whole.

I give my gratitude for the gift granted to us by the [universe/maker/your deity].

Thank you for providing me with what I need to heal.

*

Thank you for the relief and joy brought into my life by this healing herb.

It has brought me better health, better control, and a better life.

It has helped to heal me—body, mind, and soul.

Special Storage

Before we finish up this chapter, let's talk a little bit about how and where you store your product. You may just want to keep it in a medicine cupboard or on a kitchen shelf. Generally, people who use concentrated oils do this. But what I have also found is that people who use CBD flower tend to take a slightly different approach, instead giving the flower a higher status. Those who smoke either hemp or cannabis tend to develop a very close relationship with the plant itself, which is often high in reverence. Specialized containers, trays, altars, or other setups are common. The flower is given a place of honor befitting its importance to the user.

If you decide to give your CBD a place of honor in your home, the number one rule is to do what pleases you and makes you happy. I have a mirrored tray on which I place all of my herbal smoking supplies including my hemp and cannabis flowers. I have special crystal-tipped mini spoons I use only for working with my smoking herbs. I have special bowls for blending herbs and small clamp lid storage jars to keep my mixes in. I have different types of grinders. I also have an orgonite amethyst charging plate that I use to charge my flower before smoking it.

You can set up your own space any way you like (keeping oils and tinctures out of direct sunlight); do what works for you and helps you create the feeling and connection you want.

Magical Medicine

My happiest days are often the ones that take place swinging on the giant swing out by our spiritual retreat, The Spiral Labyrinth, when I have nothing to do but lie in the sun and feel the breeze on my skin as the wind pushes the swing around. These aren't the grand moments of life, but they are the moments that make every day worth waking up for. When I am out there, the connection to nature is paramount. It is a different world back in the trees, and the energy is pure, genuine, and of course, healing. The connection between myself, nature, and the divine is strong. I know my place in the universe, and it is at one.

You can find this feeling; I know you can. We all can find this connection if we but allow ourselves to. CBD can help bring you to this point in your life by helping you to heal and to see the connection between body, mind, and spirit. Cannabis provides us with magical medicine: it knows where to go, it knows what to do, and in the process, it opens our eyes and our spirit to fully heal.

CHAPTER 8

Pets

Many kinds of animals have an endocannabinoid system, so they, too, can benefit from the healing of CBD. It treats the same issues in pets that it treats in humans, including pain, inflammation, anxiety, and digestive issues. Since animals are smaller, they can use a smaller dose than humans do. I always keep a supply of 100 milligram concentrate oil on hand now for vet visits (to calm them beforehand—especially during COVID-19 quarantines when we weren't allowed into the vet office with them) or emergency situations. I had no idea how important it would be to have until we had a major emergency with no help available.

There are many ways CBD can help make your pets both healthier and happier. CBD can calm aggressive and stress-related behaviors. This is especially important in rescue animals who may have trust issues with humans or other animals. As we already know, CBD treats anxiety; this is just as true in our pets as it is in us. Car trips, vet trips, and other nervous issues can be much easier for your pet to deal with when they have CBD to help cope.

Arthritis and other forms of inflammation are just as painful to our animals as they are to us. Imagine being able to give them the same relief we can have. Well, you can! Isn't that awesome? It can be difficult to give your pet a pill every day, and pain medication can cause grogginess and organ damage along with other side effects. I think about how hard it was to get my family dog to take pain pills when I was a kid. I can imagine how much easier and much more pleasant my dog's last days alive would have been had this been available to us then. Who knows, since she died of cancer, maybe it would have given her a longer time too, but even if it didn't, I know her days would have been much more tolerable.

CBD is an antiemetic, which means it helps control vomiting, and it will also help give you an appetite. This is extremely important when animals have certain ailments. This is also why it's often used by cancer patients in chemotherapy. This prevents dehydration and malnutrition.

CBD is used to treat epilepsy and other seizure disorders in pets just as it is with humans, same as it is used to treat cancer. CBD can shrink some cancerous tumors, and of course, it helps with nausea and pain.

Cheryl's client Jacki told her experience with using CBD with their rescue dogs:

> *We rescue hospice/senior dogs that end up dumped in shelters because they are old or sick and dying. We foster them to the end so that they have the love, warmth, and grace they deserve. I started using CBD on my fosters that had cancers or other terminal illnesses. It has helped them in too many ways to even list, but they were more mobile, ate better, started to trust and love again because they weren't in so much pain. Several had tumors shrink.*

Because animals are smaller than humans (in most cases!), they do not need as big or as strong of a dose. Cheryl recommends starting with a half dropperful either by mouth or on their food. You can then increase as needed the same as you would be learning to dose yourself. For chronic issues, you can dose your pet up to three times a day. While humans can microdose themselves, animals don't get this luxury, so it is extremely important to keep a strict set schedule for when you give multiple doses throughout the day to ensure they are keeping their CBD at a steady level. For issues such as seizures, give them the CBD as soon as you can. When you know they are going to have issues—such as a trip to the vet, it's the Fourth of July and the neighbors don't care how many animals they upset with their fireworks, or other events that may be anxiety inducing—give them the dosage an hour before.

Dosage strengths for animals should start as follows:

* ★ Animals less than 20 pounds use a half dropperful of 100 mg CBD oil or 2 mg treats.

* ★ Animals 20–60 pounds use a half dropperful of 200 mg CBD oil or 5 mg treats.

* ★ Animals 60–100 pounds use a half dropperful of 300 mg oil or 10 mg treats.

* ★ Animals over 100 pounds can start with half a dropperful of 500 mg oil or 15 mg treats.

If you are giving your pet CBD on their food, be sure you aren't giving them more food than what they can eat at one time to ensure they are receiving the full dose. Leftover food in a bowl may mean a lack of CBD in the bloodstream. Animals are the same as us in that they, too, are in their best balance when CBD levels remain steady without dipping.

Cheryl's client Shannon said:

After seeing the effectiveness of CBD in humans, I could not wait to share it with my feline companion of over nine years. The taste did not bother him at all over dry or wet food. We have noticed he is more playful and happy when we use the CBD regularly. We stopped for a bit (needed to reorder), and while not drastic, the changes were there, which became more obvious how much happier he really was once we placed him back on "the good stuff." As someone

who believes our animal friends are extended family,
I am happy to treat him as such.

We know this is true for many people; our pets are our "fur babies" and keeping them in optimal health is our responsibility.

Even if you dose daily, don't forget about life's smaller occurrences that may upset your pet and require an extra dosing—nail trimming, brushing, bathing, unexpected visitors. These can all be traumatic for some animals. Giving a little more CBD can help make these moments easier on your pet and yourself.

I am thankful I now know about CBD and the benefits it has for all my animal friends—whether furry or feathered. Keeping a bottle of CBD on hand for the little ones is simply good sense.

Xena the Warrior Chicken

One late Sunday afternoon during the summer, I heard the chickens (yes, we have several we raise) making a louder-than-normal ruckus. I went outside to see what was going on, and as I rounded their fenced-in shelter, I came face to face with a Cooper's hawk pinning one of my hens to the ground outside of their pen. I was literally only a step away from this hawk clamped down on my hen's skull, trying to pull her away. I yelled, flapped my arms, and ran straight at the hawk. It let her go and flew off, first into a tree and then farther away as I kept chasing it off. I went back to pick up her motionless body. Her head was covered in blood, and she was not moving. It wasn't until I laid her down on some cardboard in the garage, I realized she was actually still breathing. I had thought she was already dead due to the amount of blood, but I wasn't going to give the hawk the satisfaction of dinner—once they know there is a food source around, they will keep coming back too, so I didn't want his kill to be successful for him.

Her breathing was incredibly shallow and uneven. Sitting watching her was torture. Her breaths were so shallow and so far apart, several times I thought she was gone, and then suddenly another gasp. We had lost a few other chickens and some ducks to the hawks over the years, but this had been the first time a hawk had not only got into the pen, but it also got a chicken out of the pen! My husband immediately went to work on securing new netting over the top of the pen. I occasionally stopped in the garage to check on the hen. From experience, I didn't think there was any way she would make it much longer, but every time I checked on her, she was still in the same nonresponsive state. I felt awful. Her legs had gone cold, so we got her a large bin, filled it with straw, and gave her a towel for a blanket. Using cotton swabs, cotton rounds, and warm water, I began cleaning all the blood off her face and head. It was slow going but she didn't seem to notice at all. There was no response from her at all. When I covered her up and tucked her in for the night, I didn't expect she would be alive in the morning. I was already surprised she had made it that long.

In the morning, she was still alive, but stiffening up considerably. I spent some more time cleaning her face and discovered the eyes we thought were gone were still in place. The swelling and bruising in her face was terrible. I knew from the amount of blood, her brain had suffered damage and was swelling. I couldn't believe she was still alive. Our previous vet had retired and the new one didn't see any type of livestock. We were at a loss for what to do. She wasn't dead, but I knew if she wasn't getting any water or food, she soon would die from dehydration or starvation for sure. So, using an eyedropper, we began giving her water mixed with baking soda, salt, and sugar—this gave her needed electrolytes. I had no idea if she was in pain or not but knew the swelling was severe around her skull, so I began giving her a dose of CBD a couple times a day. The first day of this, there was hardly any response at all. Her tongue gave a few barely noticeable flicks as the water and CBD oils were squirted in. A very small reflex, but a reflex nonetheless. We kept her partially covered with the towel to try and help keep her warm in the bin throughout the day and the next night.

The next day, she was still alive. We continued the water and CBD, and the responses from her tongue seemed to increase. By this time, we realized she wasn't going to die from the hawk attack. She had survived the worst part, but now what? She was basically comatose. I didn't want a paralyzed kind of life for her. We had no idea how badly her brain had been damaged. All we could do was keep doing what we were doing and see if things would get any better.

On the third day, they did. She began responding to our touch. When we would pick her up, she noticed. She made some movement and would open her mouth. She knew we were feeding her and was showing she was hungry. We added a gruel mixture, watering down her regular chicken feed and syringing it into her mouth, going slowly since she hadn't had any solid food for days. We continued with her water and CBD. Her legs began to regain color and warm up again.

We went from the thinned gruel to a thicker one in a spoon. We had to help her hold her head up for several days. The swelling began going down, and after a week, she opened her left eye. She was now scooting herself around in her bin and would try to stand, but her balance was way off.

She healed far faster than you or I would have with the same degree of injuries. We kept hand-feeding and helping her stand until she was able to do it on her own. Then she was able to eat on her own. Finally, after a couple of months, she did recover enough to be put back in with the rest of the flock. Her right eye sustained permanent damage in the attack, leaving her blind in that one, but we have never had a bird survive an attack before, so this was a huge accomplishment in both her healing and survival. She is a quite different chicken now compared to before. She loves humans, and due to her damaged eye, the other chickens aren't as fond of her as they used to be. She loves to follow us around, climb into laps, and swing with us on the swing. We must make sure she gets her human interaction time daily. She is the most remarkable bird I have ever encountered. Her healing was entirely unexpected and far more than I ever would have believed without seeing it myself. I am positive the CBD not only helped keep her pain minimal and helped reduce her swelling, but it sped up the healing process and made it possible for her to have the recovery she did. And yes, her name is Xena the Warrior Chicken. She earned it.

The CBD I used to save my chicken came from Cheryl's line of Fat Sam pet products named after her beloved pet. Pet parents make up a large part of her customer base, buying both oils and CBD-infused treats.

I also have three cats who use CBD. During COVID, when pets weren't allowed to have their "parents" inside with them at the vet office, a little extra dose of CBD was great to help calm their nerves, as we had several emergencies, plus a few routine visits, throughout the pandemic. Sir Gawain has liver issues, and as a recent former feral tom, his old aggressive attitude occasionally pops up, though it is less and less all the time as he is adjusting to his new indoor cat life. An extra CBD dose helps calm him down when he would rather be at the neighbor's farm chasing turkeys. Furrina takes it to help with arthritis and other pain. Morgaine, the healthiest of the bunch, is not a regular user but does take it for those vet trips.

Fat Sam

Fat Sam was Cheryl's family's dog, whom she refers to as a "foster fail" from Hurricane Katrina. After recently adopting an eight-week-old puppy from a rescue, they began wondering what was going on with the thousands of animals that had been rounded up after Katrina. With new puppy Kody in tow for a check-up, Cheryl asked the vet if he knew anything about the New Orleans rescues. He had just received fifteen dogs to go through the vetting process.

The local rescues and shelters were working together to get them into foster homes or other placements. Cheryl and her family walked down the line of cages looking at each precious face. These animals were nervous from experiencing a hurricane, being caught, sheltered, the trip from New Orleans to Chicagoland, and back at a shelter. Sam was the last in the line of cages with two other dogs. He jumped up at Cheryl as soon as he saw them, like a little kid yelling, "Pick me! Pick me!" They knew immediately they had to take him home, and so they agreed to become foster parents to him.

Foster parents bring animals to meet and greets to meet potential adopters. During Cheryl's first event, she realized after feeling defensive when anyone showed interest in Sam that Sam couldn't possibly go anywhere else. He had already found his furever home.

Loving Sam came with extra responsibilities, as he was a special needs dog with heartworms and other issues. The vet had estimated Sam's age at four when he was rescued—which means he lived to a ripe old age of nineteen. His last years were aided and improved with the CBD he took for its calming, pain-relieving, and anti-inflammatory benefits.

Cheryl said, "The resident tester of all things pumpkin and peanut butter, Fat Sam's face will be forever remembered through his CBD oils and treats specifically formulated for pets." Sam played an important role in the company as official taste tester. In his honor, CryBaby CBD also works with many local shelters and rescues.

Conclusion

First, we want to thank you for taking this journey with us. Cheryl and I both know how much CBD and hemp/cannabis have changed our lives, and we are both eager and willing to talk anyone's ear off who is ready to listen and learn about how incredible this plant really is. Relief for some, lifesaver for others, it is truly remarkable that one plant can do so much—from giving us fibers to make different materials such as cloth and plastic, to seeds for food, to cannabinoids that help our bodies work better than ever (or at least not as bad as they worked without it!).

This extremely renewable resource looks to have a bright future ahead. With a younger generation that is interested in the future of our environment and planet, cannabis is likely to play a much more important role in all its forms.

This brings me to reminding you, again, of the importance of supporting the legality of all cannabis plants to ensure everyone has equal access to medicine they may need. Those of us who have the privilege need to ensure we do the work for those who do not.

We both hope you enjoyed this book, and most importantly, we hope you learned something while reading it. I will admit, it blew my mind to see how crazy the propaganda against "marijuana" was back in the 1930s. I watched the movie *Reefer Madness* while writing *420 Meditations*. Talk about culture shock. I recommend watching it if you haven't seen it—not to try to scare you off cannabis, not by any means—but to see the absolute insanity of what the government was telling American citizens about the plant less than one hundred years ago. We need to remember, one hundred years ago is not a long time, particularly in the grand scheme of the thousands-of-years history of cannabis. We can make changes and restore it to the honor it once had. Remember, it was once the number four ingredient in medicines before Anslinger stuck his claws in. The scientific research being done shows a promising future for cannabinoids, including specialized medications.

While the science can be confusing, we tried to break it down into the simplest concepts. If you are a science buff, I highly recommend learning more about the nitty-gritty of it all. It can be quite fascinating, and with the constant research and new strides in this ever-growing field, there will always be new information to get caught up on. Having a basic grasp of the science allows you to make informed choices. Science is real, and it is your loving, happy, caring friend. Having this basic knowledge lets you know how to find out what is right for you and what isn't.

The magic begins with a seed and ends with how it can help you to heal. Remember, cannabis isn't a miracle. It was part of a divine plan, no matter what your beliefs are—whether through a god or nature, it is no mistake our bodies have an entire system made to work with the cannabinoids contained within the cannabis/hemp plant.

You are more than welcome to refer to hemp as those plants below 0.3 percent THC. I hope someday the distinction won't be necessary and we can focus on the cannabinoid content (for example, CBD cannabis) instead of trying to convince ourselves that hemp and cannabis aren't the same type of plant. Too many people do not understand the only difference is the THC count. After all, our own government didn't when they moved against "marijuana." Education will always be key, and now you can share what you have learned.

Writing this book during a global pandemic along with racial riots and an insurrection against the US government has made it extremely clear to me, if we don't begin healing as individuals first, we will never be able to heal as a nation. We must all start with ourselves. Find your connection to spirit. Live your best life with spirit.

Appendix

We have compiled this appendix for you with easy-to-access reference information to aid you on your journey.

How to Buy CBD

CBD shops are beginning to pop up across the country, but it still may be hard for many people to find a good full-service store. A full-service store will carry CBD in many forms and not only the CBD concentrate oil bottles found from gas stations to grocery stores. They may carry powdered isolates, oils, a variety of flower strains, and other products made from these ingredients.

Because CBD is legal in the United States, you are also able to order it online (flower included) and have it delivered to you. If you don't have a CBD shop near you, online is a great option.

Be sure your supplier is legit. Back in our "Science" chapter, we talked about some different ways to know if your supplier is trustworthy. Remember to ask these questions or look for this information on online stores:

1. Where was the CBD/hemp sourced from?

2. Has it been certified organic?

3. Has the CBD been tested by a third party, and are those results available to you?

These pieces of information help ensure you are getting a pure, uncontaminated product.

Where to Buy Products from This Book

Some of my favorite places to shop for products and supplies, and those who helped contribute to this book, are listed below.

* **Cheryl Cryer, CryBaby CBD,** www.crybabycbd.com (CrybabyCBD 5000 mg/30 ml full-spectrum CBD oil: https://crybabycbd.com/5000mg-cbd-oil.)

* **Lori Smerz, The Party Kitchen,** www.thepartykitchen.net

* **Krystle Hope, Crescent Sapphire,** https://www.etsy.com/shop/CrescentSapphire

* **Mountain Rose Herbs,** www.mountainroseherbs.com

- ⋆ **Sacred Smoke Herbals,**
  www.sacredsmokeherbals.com

- ⋆ **Kerri Connor,** www.kerriconnor.com

Frequently Asked Questions about CBD

We've compiled a list of the most common questions we hear while helping others navigate their wellness journey. Whether we are interacting one-on-one or in a group talk, these questions tend to pop up the most. Have additional questions? Contact us at hello@crybabycbd.com. We love to connect, collaborate, and problem solve!

What Is CBD?

Cannabidiol or CBD is one of the one hundred plus compounds (called cannabinoids) found in the aerial parts of the hemp and cannabis plants. Unlike its partner cannabinoid THC, it does not cause an intoxicating effect. CBD has the ability to act on CB1 and CB2 receptors that are part of the endocannabinoid system (ECS) in our bodies (found in all animals except insects).

Is CBD Legal?

Yes, CBD is legal if it is hemp derived and it contains less than 0.3 percent THC. The 2018 Farm Bill legalized the production and sale of hemp and its extracts.

Does CBD Get You High?

No, hemp-derived full-spectrum CBD oil has trace amounts of THC (less than 0.3 percent) but does not produce an intoxicating effect.

How Does CBD Work?

Humans and animals have CB1 and CB2 receptors that are part of a very important regulating system called the endocannabinoid system (ECS). This system, discovered in 1992 at Hebrew University, helps regulate the body's other systems, and it helps them maintain a balance known as homeostasis. The ECS receptors are located in the "brain, organs, connective tissues, glands, and immune cells."[67] When our body achieves homeostasis, it operates at optimal performance.

Along with the other one hundred plus cannabinoids, via the ECS, CBD helps regulate certain vital functions of the body, including sleep, pain, inflammation, immune, appetite, pleasure, and more.

What Are CBD's Health Benefits? How Can CBD Help Me or My Loved Ones?

Pain, insomnia, and anxiety are the most common ailments CBD is used for, but it has shown promise treating many other illnesses. It is also important to remember, new

....

67. Bradley E. Alger, "Getting High on the Endocannabinoid System," *Cerebrum* (Nov. 2013–Dec. 2013): https://www.ncbi.nlm.nih.gov /pmc/articles/PMC3997295/.

research is being done all the time, with new discoveries constantly being made.

Autoimmune disorders including MS, rheumatoid arthritis, fibromyalgia, inflammatory bowel disease (IBD: Crohn's and colitis), and diabetes have improved with regular use of CBD.

CBD reduces inflammation and supports the immune system, allowing the body's self-defense to recognize the difference between normal anatomy and foreign bodies.

Where Do I Start? Topical or Ingestible?

Customers new to CBD are often confused on where to start. We may ask a few clarifying questions to help guide you. Why are you taking it? Is it for pain? Is it for insomnia or autoimmune illnesses?

Topical: For all types of pain in a specific area (low back, neck, knee, etc.), healing irritated skin, or as part of any skincare regimen. Topical application does not enter the bloodstream.

Ingested: Tinctures, oil, gummies, tea. For insomnia, anxiety, autoimmune illness, systemic pain or inflammation, seizures, other neurological conditions, cancer, and more. Enters the bloodstream.

Inhaled: Smoked or vaped. Treats the same conditions as ingested CBD, as it also enters the bloodstream.

Inhaled is the fastest-acting method with the highest bioavailability. Sublingual is the second-fastest-acting method also with high bioavailability. Ingested is the slowest-acting method with the lowest bioavailability.

Can CBD Help My Pets?

Yes! Pets can benefit from CBD in the same way that it helps humans. It is most commonly used for pain, inflammation, and anxiety; we also see it helping pets with seizures and cancer.

Pain: Arthritis, Strain/Sprain, Overuse, Chronic Pain

Whether you're experiencing daily bodily aches, injuries from sports, or illness-related pain, you may find CBD is the natural solution you've been hoping for. Pain relief is the number one reason customers turn to CBD.

It is perfect for people who care deeply about what they put in their bodies and want an all-natural healing substance to assist with pain management instead of resorting to traditional medicine that can come with unwanted side effects.

CBD for Chronic Pain

Whether it be inflammation, back pain, joint pain, daily headaches, monthly menstrual cramps, or radiating sciatica, CBD can be a source of relief from chronic pain.

Recent literature surrounding the benefits of CBD for chronic pain has been promising. According to Upstate.edu, cannabinoids have been used in several experiments to demonstrate their effects on pain.[68]

CBD for Athletic Injuries

Many of our retail customers are active athletes, participating in high-impact sports like Roller Derby, running, or high-intensity interval training. And most of our wholesale customers are rehab and wellness centers—treating their patients' pain and injuries with the amazing, all-natural benefits of CBD.

Athletes put their bodies under immense forms of stress, which can result in pain and injury. Common injuries include sprains, tears, and even concussions. But we find that athletes are often also very health-conscious people and don't want to put chemical substances like traditional medicine into their body. For this type of individual, CBD is an alternative to explore.

But you don't have to be an athlete to reap the benefits of these medicinal properties. Whether you prefer to ingest a tincture oil or apply it topically, there are a number of CBD products that may help.

....

68. Kevin P. Hill, Matthew D. Palastro, Brian Johnson, and Joseph W. Ditre, "Cannabis and Pain: A Clinical Review," *Cannabis and Cannabinoid Research* 2, no. 1 (2017): 96–104, https://www.upstate.edu/psych/pdf/cannabispain.pdf.

Studies show that CBD oil can be a new substitute for anti-inflammatory drugs.[69] When you're working out and afterward, your muscles become inflamed, and CBD can act to put the fire out with its properties to soothe those muscles and help you naturally recover from any injuries related to exercising.

CBD for Illness-Related Pain

Individuals suffering from illness-related aches have increasingly been turning to CBD oil for natural pain management, such as:

* Fibromyalgia
* Rheumatoid arthritis
* Endometriosis
* Epilepsy
* Sleep disorders
* Multiple sclerosis
* Autoimmune diseases
* Inflammatory bowel disease (like Crohn's and others)
* Neuropathy
* Other conditions

....

69. Prakash Nagarkatti, Rupal Pandey, Sadiye Amcaoglu Rieder, Venkatesh L. Hegde, and Mitzi Nagarkatti, "Cannabinoids as Novel Anti-Inflammatory Drugs," *Future Medicinal Chemistry* 1, no. 7 (October 2009): 1333–1349, https://www.ncbi.nlm.nih.gov/pmc/articles/PMC2828614/.

If you are currently suffering from chronic pain as a result of an illness, consult your doctor. CBD may be a natural remedy to assist in your pain management plan.

How to Use CBD for Pain

There are four types or ways to use CBD products: inhale, ingest, sublingual, and topical.

The fastest way to relieve pain and inflammation is through inhalation, as this allows for the quickest route to the bloodstream. Sublingual is the second-fastest route to the bloodstream. Topicals can be used directly on the skin of the inflamed or painful area. Many CBD topicals have added essential oils and herbs to enhance the pain-relieving properties.

Anxiety/Stress/Insomnia

Many of us are challenged with stress and anxiety. Sometimes finding a balance and normal routine is disrupted by insomnia, anxiety, and agitation. We may feel the weight of work and social pressures, our health, and political tension.

And while many people self-medicate with alcohol and pills, we can probably all agree there are healthier and more natural ways to address these common ailments. This is why we offer all-natural, plant-based options as an anxiety relief alternative.

A study examining the effects of cannabidiol on anxiety-related mental health challenges came to this conclusion: "We found that existing preclinical evidence strongly supports CBD as a treatment for generalized anxiety disorder, panic disorder, social anxiety disorder, obsessive-compulsive disorder, and post-traumatic stress disorder when administered acutely."[70]

How CBD Oil Treats Anxiety

A study published on the National Center for Biotechnology Information explains that CBD interacts with serotonin receptors in a way that provides therapeutic results for our mind and body:

"Cannabis triggers a complex set of experiences in humans including euphoria, heightened sensitivity to external experience, and relaxation. The primary noneuphorizing and nonaddictive compound of cannabis, cannabidiol (CBD), has recently been shown to possess considerable therapeutic potential for treating a wide range of disorders such as chronic pain, nausea, epilepsy, psychosis, and anxiety."[71]

From a biological or chemical perspective, it's understood that CBD interacts with the endocannabinoid system

....

70. Esther M. Blessing, Maria M. Steenkamp, Jorge Manzanares, and Charles R. Marmar," Cannabidiol as a Potential Treatment for Anxiety Disorders," *Neurotherapeutics* 12 (2015): 825–836, https://doi .org/10.1007/s13311-015-0387-1.

71. Danilo De Gregorio et al., "Cannabidiol Modulates Serotonergic Transmission and Reverses Both Allodynia and Anxiety-like Behavior in a Model of Neuropathic Pain," *Pain* 160, no. 1 (January 2019): 136–150, https://www.ncbi.nlm.nih.gov/pmc/articles /PMC6319597/.

(ECS), which regulates cognitive functions, such as memory and mood, as well as pain perception.

CBD and Seizures

CBD can also be used to treat certain types of seizures. We did not touch on this in the book, as this is a therapy that requires close doctor supervision in conjunction with other pharmaceuticals. If you suffer from seizures, be sure to ask your doctor if CBD may be able to help you.

Bibliography

Alger, Bradley E. "Getting High on the Endocannabinoid System." *Cerebrum* (Nov. 2013–Dec. 2013): https://www.ncbi.nlm.nih.gov/pmc/articles/PMC3997295/.

Bennett, Chris. "Venerable Traditions: A Brief History of the Ritual and Religious Use of Cannabis." In *Cannabis and Spirituality: An Explorer's Guide to an Ancient Plant Spirit Ally*, edited by Stephen Gray, 38–58. Rochester, VT: Park Street Press, 2016.

Blessing, Esther M., Maria M. Steenkamp, Jorge Manzanares, and Charles R. Marmar. "Cannabidiol as a Potential Treatment for Anxiety Disorders." *Neurotherapeutics* 12 (2015): 825–836. https://doi.org/10.1007/s13311-015-0387-1.

Bobrow, Warren. *Cannabis Cocktails, Mocktails & Tonics: The Art of Spirited Drinks & Buzz-Worthy Libations*. Beverly, MA: Fair Winds, 2016.

Booth, Martin. *Cannabis: A History*. Transworld Digital, 2011.

Cohut, Maria. "FDA Report Evaluates CBD Product Labeling Accuracy." Medical News Today. Healthline Media. October 29, 2020. https://www.medicalnewstoday.com /articles/fda-report-evaluates-cbd-product-labeling -accuracy#CBD-content-mislabeled,-THC-not-specified.

De Gregorio, Danilo, Ryan J. McLaughlin, Luca Posa, Rafael Ochoa-Sanchez, Justine Enns, Martha Lopez-Canul, Matthew Aboud, Sabatino Maione, Stefano Comai, and Gabriella Gobbi. "Cannabidiol Modulates Serotonergic Transmission and Reverses Both Allodynia and Anxiety-like Behavior in a Model of Neuropathic Pain." *Pain* 160, no. 1 (January 2019): 136–150. https://www.ncbi.nlm.nih .gov/pmc/articles/PMC6319597/.

Deitch, Robert. *Hemp: American History Revisited: The Plant with a Divided History*. New York: Algora Pub., 2003.

Eisenstein, Toby K., and Joseph J. Meissler. "Effects of Cannabinoids on T-cell Function and Resistance to Infection." *Journal of Neuroimmune Pharmacol* 10 (2015): 204–216. https://doi.org/10.1007/s11481-015-9603-3.

Evans, Jamie. *The Ultimate Guide to CBD: Explore the World of Cannabidiol*. Beverly, MA: Fair Winds Press, 2020.

Ferrara, Mark S. *Sacred Bliss: A Spiritual History*. Lanham, MD: Rowman & Littlefield, 2018.

Gray, Stephen, ed. *Cannabis and Spirituality: An Explorer's Guide to an Ancient Plant Spirit Ally*. Rochester, VT: Park Street Press, 2017.

"Henry VIII's Reign Was a Golden Age for Hemp." Civilized, June 2, 2021, www.civilized.life/articles/henry-viii -england-hemp/.

Hill, Kevin P., Matthew D. Palastro, Brian Johnson, and Joseph W. Ditre. "Cannabis and Pain: A Clinical Review." *Cannabis and Cannabinoid Research* 2, no. 1 (2017): 96–104. https://www.upstate.edu/psych/pdf/cannabispain.pdf.

Konieczny, Eileen. *Healing with CBD: How Cannabidiol Can Transform Your Health Without the High*. With Laura Wilson. Berkeley, CA: Ulysses Press, 2018.

Leinow, Leonard, and Juliana Birnbaum. *CBD: A Patient's Guide to Medicinal Cannabis*. Berkeley, CA: North Atlantic Books, 2017.

Nagarkatti, Prakash, Rupal Pandey, Sadiye Amcaoglu Rieder, Venkatesh L. Hegde, and Mitzi Nagarkatti. "Cannabinoids as Novel Anti-Inflammatory Drugs." *Future Medicinal Chemistry* 1, no. 7 (October 2009): 1333–1349. https://www.ncbi.nlm.nih.gov/pmc/articles/PMC2828614/.

"World Timeline of Hemp." Ministry of Hemp. Accessed July 9, 2020. https://ministryofhemp.com/hemp/history/.

To Write to the Author

If you wish to contact the author or would like more information about this book, please write to the author in care of Llewellyn Worldwide Ltd. and we will forward your request. Both the author and the publisher appreciate hearing from you and learning of your enjoyment of this book and how it has helped you. Llewellyn Worldwide Ltd. cannot guarantee that every letter written to the author can be answered, but all will be forwarded. Please write to:

Kerri Connor
% Llewellyn Worldwide
2143 Wooddale Drive
Woodbury, MN 55125-2989

Please enclose a self-addressed stamped envelope for reply, or $1.00 to cover costs. If outside the U.S.A., enclose an international postal reply coupon.

Many of Llewellyn's authors have websites with additional information and resources. For more information, please visit our website at http://www.llewellyn.com.